A New Lifesty

D1453402

A COMPLETE PROGRAM FOR NATURAL CONTROL AND DRUG-FREE LIVING

NATURAL TREATMENTS FOR

HYPERTENSION

AGATHA THRASH, M.D. & CALVIN THRASH, M.D.

Contents

Preface

In the 1994 edition of Harrison's Principles of Internal Medicine, Dr. Gordon H. Williams calls hypertension "the most important public health problem in developed countries."

A common, yet puzzling problem in our contemporary society, hypertension is no respecter of age or sex. Physicians generally tell their patients to take medication, limit physical activity and learn to live with it. But can we rely on a drug to correct hypertension? Is taking a drug an "easy" way out, or is it filled with the potential for creating worse health problems in the future? Are the significant known side-effects, as well as potiential unknown ones, acceptable, even if the medication actually brings blood pressure down? This book will answer these questions as well as discuss how to treat high blood pressure at home. No one should be unaware of the cause, course or treatment of high blood pressure.

You can buy at a health food store or pharmacy your own blood pressure cuff and stethoscope to follow the response you make to the remedies described in this book. Chances are very good that you, along with thousands of others can learn to control your blood pressure yourself, without using dangerous medications which are hazardous to your health.

It is estimated that more than 65 million Americans suffer from high blood pressure to some degree. It has been called the "Silent Killer" for good reason. High blood pressure affects adversely the heart, as a major risk factor for heart attacks and a prominent cause of enlarged hearts leading to congestive heart failure. The blood vessels are damaged, tremendously increasing the risk of strokes, hardening of the arteries, and permanent damage of the kidneys and the retinas. And it is largely "silent," since there are few if any symptoms that can be relied upon as an indicator of high blood pressure.

Whereas older physicians taught that elevated systolic pressure alone, without diastolic hypertension, was largely innocuous, we now know that this is not the case. In males who have a diastolic blood pressure of 82 or less, but a systolic pressure of 158 or greater, the risk of cardiovascular mortality is increased by two and one-half times (250%).

Hypertension increases the risk of complications of other diseases. Atrial fibrillation also increases your risk of getting a stroke. If you add hypertension to an already existing case of atrial fibrillation, you will triple your risk of strokes above that of one without atrial fibrillation. Atherosclerosis increases your risk of Alzheimer's disease. Add hypertension for many years and the risk increases. Diabetes increases your risk of getting eye diseases resulting in blindness. If you add hypertension to your diabetes, you double your likelihood of going blind. [132,133]

In the past, the great preponderance of high blood pressure was termed "essential hypertension," indicating that it was of unknown cause. But in recent years, it has become increasingly apparent that high blood pressure - like coronary heart disease, non-insulin dependent diabetes, and even cancer - is actually a lifestyle disease with a constellation of factors contributing to it from an unhealthful lifestyle. In this book we will discuss many of these factors, and what can be done to help to control the hypertension plaguing our nation.

section
one

defining the scope of hypertension

2

Case History

The following case illustrates how hypertension is often a part of a picture of general metabolic disease. The scope of hypertension is quite broad, but the treatment can be often simple as is illustrated here.

RB, a 68 year old white man living near Atlanta, Georgia had become house bound voluntarily and a cardiac cripple because of his physical problems. He was a former employee of the city of Atlanta and had been friends with the men at the fire station nearest his home, where he got his blood pressure taken about once a week. Although he was a very religious man, RB had stopped going to church one year before because of fear he would die in church and require removal "feet first." His daughter had been my patient for many years and requested me to go with her to see her father in his home. He received me graciously, and had all 17 bottles of his medications on a small tray for me to see the adequacy of his treatment from his doctor. He was taking medicine for angina (chest pain on exertion), hypertension (three medicines), sleeplessness, a peptic ulcer he had had since World War II, mild diabetes, arthritis and recurring headaches. He was very faithful in taking his medicines, but said he never felt strong, nor was he ever "himself" but guessed he was just old and "worn out."

I told him that as healthy as I was I would not feel good if I took all those medicines. I suggested he come for a patient session at Uchee Pines Health Conditioning Center to see if we could help him.

His blood pressure even with all his medicines was 172/93. He said that level was not bad, as it often ran 215/108. Although it was a hot June day, he refused to remove his jacket during the drive to Uchee Pines as the wind on his chest might cause a heart attack. His daughter said he believed he would die in December, the first anniversary of his wife's death of

4   *breast cancer. Although only 5' 10" he weighed in at 196 pounds. His fasting blood sugar was 111.*

We began his treatment at once: a soak in a nice warm bathtub; a salt and oil-free vegetarian diet without dairy or eggs, and a stroll with his lifestyle counselor. He returned after a 10-minute rest, a distance of about one city block. We gave him hawthorn berry tea in 10 glasses of water daily. We stopped his nitroglycerine, both skin patches and long-acting pills; he insisted on keeping the sublingual tablets "in case of emergency." His diabetes came under control after one day of fasting and a weight loss of five pounds. Within three weeks he had taken himself off all other medication with our assistance except for some chloral hydrate which he had taken for twenty years for sleeping. He was a new man. He went back home eager to work in his yard and plant some vegetables. He began going to church and out to eat at the salad bar of a local vegetarian restaurant with a "lady friend." He has now passed nine anniversaries of his wife's death and is still going strong at 77. "The boys at the fire department" keep up with his blood pressure, and his local internist thinks he is a miracle with a drug-free blood pressure around 130/78-82. His daughters are very grateful.

what is hypertension?

Definition of hypertension

Hypertension can be defined as an increase in the tension on blood vessels, primarily the very smallest arteries. This tension is caused by many factors, some of which are hereditary, some due to pressure from surrounding tissue, while others are lifestyle or emotional. When these factors contribute to a blood pressure reading higher than considered healthful, it is called hypertension.

Blood pressure is defined as the pressure put on the blood by the combined forces of heartbeat, weight of the substances like iron or calcium carried in the blood, flow characteristics, and external pressure applied to the blood vessels. This pressure is exerted by clothing, tissue pressure, and muscle tone. Blood pressure can be measured by simple equipment--a blood pressure apparatus and a stethoscope.

There are two levels usually observed: systolic and diastolic. The systolic is the higher of the two and is made by the actual pressure from the heart to pump the blood. The diastolic is the pressure made by the muscles of the blood vessels themselves, during the time the heart is refilling and the valves are closed--the so-called "resting pressure." Since

6   the cardiovascular system is a closed circuit of vessels, pressure in it never drops to zero.

When only the systolic blood pressure is elevated in older people it is the result of structural changes occurring with aging. These changes include decreased connective tissue elasticity and hardening of the arteries, which in turn cause increased resistance of blood vessels to the passage of blood. There is also diminished nerve sensitivity as people grow older, leading to a decline in smooth muscle relaxation.[1] This type of hypertension should be treated only if very high, and can be successfully treated in many patients, by the use of simple measures.

In 1992, the National Institutes of Health issued guidelines for typical adults with systolic blood pressure above 130, or diastolic blood pressure above 85. This represented a new definition of hypertension, different from that established by the American College of Cardiologists (ACC). The ACC had established 140/90 to be the beginning of abnormality. This new definition represented a step in a right direction, as we believe 120/80 to be the upper limit of ideal.

In 1979, a study showed that of adult men having a systolic (first) reading from 138-147 there is a 36% higher chance of early death, and women have a 22% higher risk than normals. With systolic readings from 148-157, men have a 68% greater than normal risk of early death, and women have a 35% greater risk. These percentages are greater than either group would have been expected to have at systolic readings of 120 or less.[2]

The American Heart Association journal named *Hypertension* reported in early September of 1992 that cases of hypertension treated with drug medication could lead to nerve atrophy and shrinkage of the brain. It is not so much the portion of the brain we call "grey matter" that shrinks, but the white matter, the part enabling one to quite easily communicate from one part of the brain to another. Thus, dexterity, both physically and mentally, might be retarded by longstanding high blood pressure.

In 1992 *Science News* reported a definition of Stage I (mild) hypertension as 140/90 to 159/99; Stage II (moderate) as 160/100 to 179/109. Stage III (severe) would then be anything above 180/110. [3]

Even mild hypertension boosted mortality in persons followed over a 20 year period in the famous Framingham Heart Study. Levels no higher than 140 to 159 have significance if the person is over age 60 at the time of initial diagnosis. [4]

Ideally, blood pressure should remain the same throughout life when no other kind of disease develops. The "normal" aging process should not be accompanied by a rise in blood pressure. [5] So, why then do so many of us see an increase in blood pressure along with an increase of our years?

Why does blood pressure rise with age? In the United States it has been found that children have twice the risk of developing high blood pressure if either of their parents are hypertensive. Stress, which has become a nearly unavoidable part of everyday American life, has been found to be an important factor in the development of high blood pressure, as have weight gain and diet. The standard Western custom of eating which includes overeating, the use of meats, refined foods (especially the fats, sugars, and other very highly refined carbohydrates), dairy products, between meal snacks, alcohol, coffee and soft drinks, puts a person in a high risk category for hypertension. [6] Emotional temperament, chilling of the extremities, noises, lack of exercise and certain drugs can also have an influence on the blood pressure.

In studies done on native people living in the Solomon Islands, where the Western diet and fast-paced way of lifestyle are unknown, there also appeared to be no high readings of blood pressure. In some groups on the islands, there was not even an increase in the level of their blood pressure with age. [7]

8   It is assumed that their various hereditary factors, and a much calmer lifestyle with their positive attitudes toward life were the elements that preserved their blood pressure.

Identify hypertension risk factors early in life Hypertension risk factors can be identified early in life before the outward signs of any disease are present. If these factors are recognized, precautions can be taken, with non-drug programs of treatment.[8] The treatments are made up of lifestyle changes including changes in diet and sedentary habits.

Many physicians have resigned themselves to the belief that there are no effective means of preventing or delaying the onset of hypertension. But this is not true, for it is well-known in research circles that a vegetarian diet will delay or prevent the onset of high blood pressure, or will control it in most patients once it has been diagnosed.[9] Part of this conflict is caused by a reluctance on the part of physicians to recommend changes in lifestyle as their patients might consider them to be meddlers, or that their "recommendations are practically pious."[10] Few doctors want to be thought of as "pious" and so take the face-saving route of prescribing drugs.

There is much conflict of thought in the medical community over this issue. Prolonged life has been found by some investigators from reducing blood pressure with medications; but in other studies proof that a drug approach to hypertension is safe or prolongs life was not found. Some studies even reveal a shorter lifespan for people who use hypertension medications. Nevertheless, an elevation of blood pressure should not be neglected just because one is not planning to use drugs. There are effective natural ways to treat high blood pressure.

Nowadays, many physicians will recommend non-drug approaches to a patient who refuses drug therapy.[11] With instruction and physician support, patients become willing to take preventive measures on their own.[12] Because it is the patients who stand to lose the most by not adopting preventive measures, it is to their benefit to learn about prevention and apply the knowledge.

The patient is quite fortunate whose physician will take the time to educate him or her on the causes and the natural ways of managing blood pressure, instead of merely putting a cap (prescribing drugs) on signs and symptoms of this potentially explosive condition.[13] Many patients treated with drugs will begin to experience deteriorating health and eventually their quality of life will decline. They are then susceptible to many different types of diseases, both those affecting the immune system and those affecting the heart. It is a greater service to patients to give instructions on curing their entire physical condition with diet and exercise. The practice of lifestyle change can be enjoyable and even exciting when approached with a spirit of discovery, and the rewards make every effort and attention to detail highly worthwhile. Drugs will not cure the person, rather they will add metabolic stresses. The ill effects of drugs will be discussed in a later section.

Some patients will respond 100% to any method of treatment, but no single method of treatment will be effective with all individuals. The reasons for this may have to do with the genetic, psychological and physical factors involved in the maintenance of blood pressure. But by following the lifestyle changes suggested in this book, most patients with high blood pressure will respond with a return to normal blood pressure readings and improved health in general.

10

summary of major ideas and treatments

The following pages give a brief summary of all major matters covered in this book. It has been prepared for the convenience of the person who would like to see an overview of the book, or wants a quick reference for something read in the book. We believe this summary will make the book a "user friendly" book for its size and generous technical and scientific content. This summary does not, however, take the place of reading the full text. We substantiate and amplify the summary items in the main body of the book.

We suggest that you have a pen and paper near at hand as you read this chapter. Jot down any notation you read which could be applicable to your health or situation. Then, as you read the book, make more extended notes if you choose, and explanations for you to review from time to time to keep the reasons for your treatments and for the lifestyle changes fresh in mind. In this way you can keep your resolutions sharpened and your will constantly firm. The cause: of failure of

12   the simple remedies for hypertension in most instances is slipping gradually, step by step, back into the lifestyle which has caused the hypertension. The changes must be permanent. Therefore you must put forth the effort to make those adjustments that will make you enjoy living healthfully. People like the kind of cooking they grew up with. If you had grown up in a country where they have no hypertension, chances are almost 100% that you would like that kind of lifestyle. You can learn to like it now! Many old dogs have been taught new tricks. Believe that!

Summary notations

Buy your own blood pressure cuff and stethoscope to take blood pressure readings in your home--avoid "whitecoat hypertension."

The best general program is the Health Recovery Program in Chapter Nine.

Drugs are not the best answer to essential hypertension and can actually shorten life even though the blood pressure comes down. The drugs used can promote heart attacks, impotence, memory loss, cancer and other serious illnesses.

Massage, back rubs and foot rubs are very beneficial to bring the blood pressure down. The effects are only temporary but useful.

Warm baths and saunas are good for the blood pressure, but only temporarily. They should be used when the blood pressure is likely to go up from stress.

Avoid hormonal drugs and excess salt during pregnancy because they increase the risk of hypertension in the children on maturing. See "Tips to Reduce Sodium Intake" in Chapter Seven, page 63.

Risk of strokes from any cause can be reduced by daily eating 10-15 walnut halves or half a cup of cooked soybeans.

The person with essential hypertension would do well to *treat the disease as one would treat diabetes*, since the hereditary causes for hypertension are the same in many people as for diabetes. Cut out sugar, free fats, heavy proteins and salt until the blood pressure is in normal range and stable, and always afterward severely restrict these foods in the diet. See Chapter Seven, page 61, for more details.

Moderate exercise after meals will increase blood flow to skeletal muscles and cause blood pressure to drop.

Hypertension can be caused by too little or no exercise, emotional tension, inborn metabolic error and low dietary magnesium and calcium.

When *sudden stresses* or trials beset us, the blood pressure immediately goes up, if only to a very small degree. Neutralize stress with exercise.

Hostility is associated with greater diastolic readings (second number in the blood pressure reading). Learn to pray and develop the peaceful spirit of Heaven.

Correct all *problems in your social contacts* and emotional expressions. See Chapters Five and Six for discussion.

Reorganize your home life and make changes where necessary (see Chapter Six).

Learn to avoid tense conversations. Be "laid back." Analyze all stresses and learn to handle them. See Chapter Five on stress.

Remember that exercise neutralizes stress. Bear in mind that overeating is a form of biochemical stress.

Avoid annoying noises. Any way you can reduce noise in your workplace will reduce tensions on your muscles and lower blood pressure.

Always keep your arms and legs warm. During cold weather there is an overall increase in blood pressure readings in doctors' offices.

Drink plenty of water. Increase water drinking to at least eight glasses per day. This can include caffeine-free herb teas, but no caffeinated or decaffeinated coffees, teas, colas or chocolate, and no fruit juice between meals.

14   When a person who has been diagnosed with a higher than normal pulse rate does not *stay physically fit*, his or her blood pressure is more likely to rise.

Eat more fresh fruits and vegetables and less food in general. Training the appetite to accept less food will frequently have a noticeable effect on the blood pressure.

Cut out salt, whether added at the factory or in the home, for a trial period of four months and see the results. See "Tips to Reduce Sodium Intake" in Chapter Seven, page 63.

As the *intake of fiber*, potassium, calcium and magnesium goes up in the diet, blood pressures go down. Keep boron, copper and chromium levels up and iron and tyramine down. See Appendix for the important actions and food sources of these and other nutrients.

Three large stalks of celery ground in a blender yield about a glassful of puree. This amount taken daily for three months gave a 13% reduction in blood pressure in one study conducted on a group of hypertensives.

Two tablespoons of freshly ground flaxseed taken with a meal may have a beneficial effect on blood pressure.

Garlic and onion have been shown to benefit some people who have high blood pressure.

Uric acid is a waste product from foods high in purines, food substances related to protein. *When uric acid is high in the blood it can raise blood pressure.* See Appendix for listing of foods high in purines.

Avoid free fats (margarine, mayonnaise, fried foods, cooking fats, salad oils and peanut butter) because they raise the blood pressure in most susceptible persons.

Learn never to overeat. Overeating, even of healthful foods, increases the likelihood that blood pressure will go up. It stimulates the adrenals and raises the blood pressure.

Eating pork, even unsalted, may cause high blood pressure as it is high in purines, sodium, and other harmful factors.

Allergies of various kinds can raise blood pressure. You should undertake an "Elimination and Challenge" diet to discover foods that may have an effect on your blood pressure. See Chapter Nine, page 95, for information on how to do this test.

The most favorable diet for people with high blood pressure is a simple vegan diet--fruits, vegetables, whole grains and a few nuts and seeds. Breakfast should be principally fruit and whole grains and lunch should be mainly vegetables and whole grains. Either or both meals can have one or two tablespoons of nuts.

Fruit, either raw or preserved in some way other than with salt, vinegar or sugar, has been found to help people with high blood pressure or increased uric acid. Fill your breakfast menu with fruit and reduce the quantity of other foods-- breads, cereals, etc.

Overweight, particularly of the abdomen or trunk, is related to hypertension. Diet, exercise, weight control and a support group to help you stay with the program, can help put an end to hypertension.

Exercise, vigorous but not violent, is of enormous benefit to most patients, particularly for hypertensive adolescents.

Avoid dressing in scant clothing while exercising because it promotes chilling of the extremities and overheating of the trunk. The great contrast in blood temperature may trigger a fatal heart rhythm disturbance in those with already sick hearts. Further, those particles in the blood called platelets that promote blood clotting become more sticky with contrasting temperatures in the bloodstream.

The benefits of exercise as a treatment for hypertension begin immediately and will have after-exercise advantages even before a state of physical fitness is attained.

Practice abdominal breathing. For the method and a discussion, see Chapter Ten, page 102.

Start a program of exercise today which you are certain

16 will not harm you. We suggest walking, gardening, etc. Isometric exercises are quite helpful. Running in place and trampoline workouts are useful also.

Control your weight. See Chapter Eleven for a complete weight control program. On the paragraphs following are a summary of ideas.

Cut out all free fats completely (butter, margarine, mayonnaise, fried foods, cooking fats, salad oils, peanut butter and all other nut and seed butters). You will not miss the nutrients, your set point for weight will come down, and your hypertension will be benefited on a diet free of all visible fats. You can still use a few nuts and seeds. See discussion in Chapter Eleven for reasons.

Change your cuisine. The less you eat meat, milk, eggs and cheese, the more weight you will lose. The most favorable diet for weight loss is a vegetarian diet of only fruits, vegetables, whole grains, nuts or seeds.

Eat nothing after three in the afternoon. The metabolism changes at about 3:00 p.m. to storage rather than production gear. The more raw foods you eat, the better it will be for weight loss.

Immediately after meals take some exercise out-of-doors for about 25 minutes. It should not be strenuous, but should be brisk or moderate. Mild to moderate exercise actually promotes digestion.

The smaller the variety of food eaten at one meal, the lower the set point for weight. More weight will be gained from a 600 calorie meal containing ten different dishes made from complex recipes, than a 600 calorie meal containing only two or three simple dishes plus bread and spread.

Fasting is good for the blood pressure. If you do not take medicines which require food to be taken with it, leave off all food beginning after breakfast one day--skipping lunch and supper that day, all food the next day, and breaking the fast with a small breakfast on the next morning.

Fasting is a beneficial way to gain appetite control, to

help accustom yourself to the tastes of different foods, to restore function of insulin receptors and to help lose weight.
(See Chapter Eleven for full information.)

Herbs have been used for centuries in the treatment of
every human ill. Although they are only beginning to be rediscovered by conventional physicians, herbs are an effective
and harmless therapy when used properly. Unlike drugs, they
generally cause no injurious or disturbing side effects, and
their proper use will not lead to further illness or death.

Useful teas for lowering blood pressure are the diuretic
herbs--watermelon seed, dandelion, cornsilk, buchu, burdock
and uva ursi. Use one to two cups, four times per day. [127]

Hawthorn berry and black cohosh, anti-inflammatory and
muscle relaxant herbs, are also excellent teas for reducing
blood pressure. Yarrow and mistletoe are also good for blood
pressure. Drink four cups of any of these teas in one day. Tea
must be made fresh daily to be effective, and only from herbs
that were harvested less than one year from the time they are
used (see Chapter Twelve for details). To slow the heart rate,
use lily of the valley tea. Although lily of the valley
(*convallaria majolis*) is listed as a toxic herb, it has been used
for centuries for heart problems. We have found it to be generally free of side effects in moderate usage, such as a cupful
of the infusion of the leaves 1-3 times daily. Nevertheless, it
should be used with care, and preferably under the supervision and monitoring of your healthcare provider. It should
not be used in conjunction with cardiac or blood pressure
drugs.

Hydrotherapy is one of the most effective ways of temporarily treating acutely elevated blood pressure. It should
be used when the patient is under stress or has a sharp rise in
blood pressure.

A hot foot bath lowers the blood pressure as does a 20-
90 minute neutral (95-100 degrees) or hot (100-110 degrees)
bath. Caution should be used when stepping into the water,

18 especially when it is very hot. The blood pressure can go up temporarily within the first 20-60 seconds if there is an extreme change in temperature.

Fomentations (hot compresses or hot wet towels) can also be used to bring blood pressure down. (See Chapter Twelve for details.)

Avoid alcohol like the plague. Its damaging effect hits not only the brain but every cell it touches, heart, kidneys and blood vessels. Many reports link the use of any kind of alcoholic drink to elevation of blood pressure.

For most human beings, exercise alone does not reverse high blood pressure. We also need to *reduce salt, weight, stress, sugar and alcohol.* These may all cause insulin resistance, a prominent cause of high blood pressure. (See Chapter Three.)

Elevated insulin levels and insulin resistance can occur in people with normal blood sugar levels from eating highly refined carbohydrates such as white rice, white flour, pastries, white bread, honey or sugar, or eating between meals.

Swelling of the feet and ankles will go down on a diet similar to the one we give for diabetics, as the metabolic cause of hypertension and diabetes is shared by many with high blood pressure. In both diseases we find sodium buildup in cells and fluid retention.

basic causes of hypertension

Where does hypertension begin?   Are there any organs of the body we can say are more involved in causing hypertension than any other, as wrong functioning of the thyroid causes hyperthyroidism and wrong functioning of the nerves causes multiple sclerosis? Yes! Apparently the pancreas and the kidneys, along with the liver and muscles, are more involved in producing what we call essential hypertension than any other organs. In the process, a hormone is produced which we have always looked on as being uniformly beneficial--insulin. But research has revealed that insulin can cause injury when it circulates in the blood in too great quantity. The pancreas puts out too much insulin in a condition called insulin resistance. This condition is caused by lifestyle factors which we will discuss later.

Hypertension, overweight, high blood cholesterol and triglycerides, and diabetes are all related to overproduction of insulin.

Getting at the cause   Essential hypertension is the name given by doctors to high blood pressure not caused by a

20 known condition such as kidney disease, a brain tumor, over-whelming stress, etc. For decades we have said essential high blood pressure has no known cause. Yet we have recognized that essential hypertension tends to occur in families also having diabetes.

Hypertension linked to gene Scientists have recently linked essential hypertension with a gene.[28] This same gene also appears to make a person more susceptible to diabetes, heart disease, obesity of the trunk and cancer. A number of doctors in the past few decades have noticed this susceptibility in hypertensive patients or close relatives of the patients. Other related problems include elevated blood cholesterol and triglycerides, and pancreatic cancer.[29, 30, 31] This association of disorders has been dubbed "Syndrome X."

Since approximately 1970, it has been found that people who have this group of familial diseases have too much insulin in their blood. Yet their blood sugar levels are not as low as we would think they should be, but are usually somewhat high. One large study demonstrated that in patients with hypertension, there was both increased insulin secretion by the pancreas, and decreased insulin sensitivity of body cells.[32] These patients are said to be insulin resistant, and the disorder has been called "Insulin Resistance Syndrome" or "Hyperinsulinism." This disorder is characterized by the patient's inability to respond to normal insulin levels and the need to produce far too much insulin in order to keep the blood sugar normal. It has been noted, that among patients with hypertension, more than half are insulin resistant. Insulin can be said to "irritate" body cells and produce these diseases.

The high blood cholesterol seen in patients with this syndrome has been a particular pattern of high levels of low density cholesterol—the injurious kind—and low levels of high density cholesterol—the healthful kind. The triglycerides have been usually elevated also.

Dr. Ralph DeFronzo, Professor of Medicine at the University of Texas in San Antonio, commenting on the wide-spread occurrence of this condition says that 80% of people who visit a doctor's office have one of three disorders:

Obesity. One of three people in the United States is at least 30 pounds overweight.

Type II diabetes. The adult form of the disease. This represents five to ten percent of the population of America.

High blood pressure. One out of five people in the United States has high blood pressure.

There are specific mechanisms within our bodies, which when not working properly lead to insulin resistance. Most cells in the body have thousands of tiny receptors for insulin on the surface which cannot be seen with a microscope. To give an illustration of what these receptors are like, imagine little docking stations which insulin will

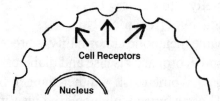

Artist's conception of "docking station" cell receptors

slide into as it floats by in the blood stream. The insulin is taken into the cell, along with glucose (blood sugar), which has attached itself to the insulin molecule. The glucose is converted into an energy storage molecule called adenosine triphosphate, or ATP. Approximately 1/3 of our glucose is oxidized into ATP for energy and the remaining 2/3 is converted into glycogen, the storage form of sugar in animals, that corresponds to starch in plants. In diabetics, hypertensives, overweight and coronary patients, there is a defect in this glycogen synthetic pathway.

As people get older, these conditions become more severe. By the age of 70, one out of four people is diabetic

22 (25%), one out of two is obese (50%), and one out of two has high blood pressure (50%).

In insulin resistance the process of conversion of glycogen to glucose is impaired. A process inside the liver and muscles is responsible for this main abnormality of insulin resistance. In insulin resistance, sodium inside cells, especially muscle cells, is thought to be the fundamental underlying abnormality. This leads to heightened reactivity of the muscle cells, especially to stress,[33] causing hypertension. This same metabolic abnormality is present in all high blood pressure, coronary disease and diabetes.

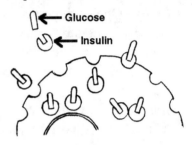

The ideal is just enough insulin, just enough glucose (none to spare), but plenty of the shallow receptors so that insulin, attached to glucose, can readily back into the cell, as a truck backs into a factory to bring fuel.

Women risk another danger from insulin resistance. Those women with increased insulin in the blood have a significantly higher risk of breast cancer whether or not they are overweight or have large breasts.[34] In one study, the more fat women lost from the abdomen (not general loss or loss of fat from other areas) the more their blood pressure dropped.

It has been demonstrated that blood pressure increases on a sugar rich diet.[35] The reason for this is the development of insulin resistance by body cells with resulting high levels of insulin in the blood. Hypertension developed on the high sugar diet, but could be successfully treated by exercise or removing sugar from the diet.[36]

For most human beings, exercise alone does not lower mild high blood pressure. We also need to cut down the total number of calories in the diet, reduce weight, salt, sugar, stress and alcohol.[37]

Extra insulin is manufactured to compensate for this loss of insulin effectiveness. As insulin resistance increases and the surplus insulin continues to circulate in increasing levels in the blood, the pancreas is forced to work excessively hard. At this point, certain factors like severe stresses from infection, overweight, lack of exercise, advancing age, as well as eating too much, excessive use of fats, sugar, and protein and all manner of refined grains and carbohydrates, could cause the pancreas to be unable to produce enough insulin to keep the blood sugar in a normal range. A diagnosis of diabetes must now be made!

Beta cells in the pancreas are programmed to respond instantly with extra insulin to increases in blood sugar. ATP, the energy molecule, is required for all chemical

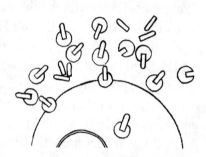

Insulin resistance is the condition of producing, but not properly utilizing a normal or even increased amount of insulin, combined with the inability to take up and use glucose properly. The cells can only respond sluggishly to insulin, because there are only two places shown here for insulin to use to escort sugar into the cell.

processes in the body. Because the pancreas is overworked, either from continued overeating or deterioration of the general condition, it can fail quite suddenly. Then, since there is not enough insulin being produced by the pancreas, glucose cannot be converted into high energy ATP. The condition then produced is Type II diabetes; insulin resistance is the first step in this development. These processes are the reason why diabetics often don't feel well and lack normal amounts of energy.

Interesting Genetic Features People with Type I, or juvenile diabetes, who need to take insulin injections have some increased risk of high blood pressure and heart attacks.

24 This is because the excess injected insulin has a similar effect in the body to excess natural insulin produced by the pancreas. The person with Type I diabetes should strive to use the smallest amount of insulin possible. To adequately control blood sugar, eating extra food or a sweet treat and "covering it with a shot" is a dangerous practice and should never be indulged.

Even self-produced excess insulin in the bloodstream causes blood fat disturbances in the following ways:

1. Excess insulin interferes with proper levels of the blood fats VLDL*, IDL*, LDL* and HDL*. These are blood fats which are dangerous in large concentrations, except for HDL (high density lipoprotein). VLDL (very low density lipoprotein) is synthesized by the liver. This process is controlled by insulin and when insulin levels go up, more VLDL is produced. As VLDL is processed in the body, it becomes IDL (intermediate density lipoprotein). The enzyme, lipoprotein lipase, is the catalyst for this process. IDL is one of the most atherogenic particles found in the body and is in high concentration in all insulin-resistant states. IDL is then converted to LDL, leaving a pure cholesterol core and pure apo-B100. This explains why the cascade of blood fat disturbances seen in Type II diabetes and obesity with hypertension have hyperinsulinemia as the root cause. Unfortunately, by this same mechanism, high density lipoprotein (HDL) which needs to be high, is lowered.

2. The major blood fat disturbances in Type II diabetes are not caused by high blood cholesterol, but by a decrease in HDL and an increase in triglycerides. These are the two major disturbances most associated with high blood insulin.

Surplus insulin also activates the sympathetic nervous

---

*Very Low, Intermediate, Low Density & High Density Lipoproteins system. This is the primary link between increased insulin in the blood and essential hypertension.

The effect of excess insulin on the nerves, specifically sympathetic nervous system, will raise blood pressure because the sympathetic nervous system is in charge of the "fight or flight" reaction, speeding up the pulse rate and increasing norepinephrine (a hormone of the sympathetic nervous system).

In one study it was found that injecting insulin into the vein of a person's forearm caused norepinephrine release in the forearm to be threefold greater in hypertensives, than in normal subjects.[42] This indicates the already present genetic mechanism for hypertension built into people whose families have hypertension.

Fasting or significant restriction of calories will suppress the sympathetic nervous system activity while overeating will stimulate it. Refined carbohydrates and fats both stimulate the sympathetic nervous system even when the total calorie intake is not excessive. When people overeat, especially refined carbohydrates and fats, their metabolism goes up. An increased metabolism stimulates the sympathetic nervous system to cause hypertension.

Dr. Lewis Landsburg, Professor of Medicine at the University of Pennsylvania, writes on the subject of insulin resistance and comments, "Insulin is a signal that permits the brain to assess nutritional status and adjust sympathetic nervous system outflow accordingly." This is similar to a feedback mechanism. Dr. Landsburg believes that insulin resistance in overweight people may be a compensatory mechanism aimed at increasing the metabolic rate. The body hopes, so to speak, that the excess insulin will stabilize the weight and help prevent further obesity. But the excess insulin acts on the kidneys to increase sodium and fluid retention, and sympathetic stimulation of blood vessels which increases blood pressure.

It is estimated that up to 25% of people who are not

26 overweight in America inherit or acquire insulin resistance. Stated another way, the person who has inherited insulin resistance, who is neither overweight, nor hypertensive and is not Type II diabetic, has a 25% chance of becoming insulin resistant. Avoiding obesity in this case does not prevent insulin resistance or sympathetic nervous system stimulation, and the result will probably be high blood pressure. For these persons, the best kind of treatment is daily exercise, a day or two each week of fasting, being careful never to overeat even though it does not lead to overweight, and being regular in all health habits. The herbal remedies will also be helpful.

The Framingham study, an investigation that has been on-going for over 30 years in Massachusetts, found that lean people with high blood pressure were more likely to become obese over the next 11 years than were normal people, apparently because of the excess insulin they produce.

For people with high blood pressure, whether they are overweight or not, Dr. Landsburg states that treatment strategies directed at trying to decrease insulin resistance and sympathetic nervous system stimulation are sound physiologically. He also found that non-drug therapies such as salt restriction, eating less food, doing physical exercise, and omitting the supper meal and between-meal-eating, as well as weight reduction programs if needed, play an important role in reducing insulin resistance and high blood pressure.

Insulin levels in the blood are measured by first checking a fasting blood sugar level, then giving the patient a large meal. Blood sugar and insulin levels are checked at one hour and two hours after the meal is eaten. Blood sugar levels may be found to be entirely normal or only mildly elevated, but the blood insulin levels will be abnormally high when insulin resistance is present.

Obese patients with normal glucose tolerance tests, as well as those with Type II, adult-onset diabetes, who already have abnormal glucose tolerance tests, can both have the same degree of insulin resistance. The difference between them is quite distinct. The insulin secretion from the pancreas in a person with diabetes is still high, but it has begun to decline and can no longer overcome the insulin resistance of the cells. But an overweight person without diabetes still may be able to produce more than enough insulin to force the passage of sugar from the blood into the cells. When the pancreas fails, diabetes is then diagnosed.

A **total-vegetarian diet** is the best one for recovery from high blood pressure. Even though more bulk is eaten and appetite is satisfied, there are generally far less calories taken in. For example, compare 100 calories of fruit and 100 calories in a milk chocolate bar. The Hershey Bar is higher in certain forms of sugar that are absorbed very quickly, causing the blood sugar to rise rapidly. When the blood sugar rises so quickly, it often soars higher than normal. A high blood sugar by itself can cause injury to the interior of the blood vessels, creating a higher risk for hardening of the arteries with resulting hypertension. But when you eat a whole fruit with naturally occurring sugar and fiber in it, even though the total amount of sugar is the same as in the Hershey Bar, the blood sugar rises slowly, is absorbed efficiently and tapers off quickly. It is easy to see that **the type of food eaten** makes a difference to the working of the pancreas, and not just the quantity of calories from sugars which the food contains.

It also makes a difference **when you eat**. Eating between meals and at night overworks the pancreas. The pancreas needs a rest between meals to rejuvenate itself. If it is kept working all day with repeated small meals, each of which calls for a load of insulin, after several years it can become exhausted and unable to put out sufficient insulin. This condition, which is critical, is diagnosed as diabetes. But the situation is not a sudden event, it has been building up for years.

When **sugar and fat intakes are kept low**, and the blood

28 pressure comes down and stabilizes, a person can expect no more problems with high blood pressure, even though he may have genetic or other abnormalities present.

Causes of Insulin Resistance. The causes of insulin resistance vary. **Aging** is one cause. Beginning usually at about age 20, there is an increase in insulin resistance with each decade.

A second cause is genetics. Some people have a definite hereditary predisposition to insulin resistance. These are the same people who have an hereditary predisposition to hypertension. If insulin levels are measured in children at the age of two years, a prediction can be made as to who will become diabetic. If high insulin levels are found, these children will almost certainly become Type II diabetics and more prone to hypertension and early heart attacks unless great care is employed to control lifestyle and weight. When insulin levels are evaluated in any one of several conditions--fasting, one-hour after eating or two-hours after eating--they will also predict who will be likely to have myocardial infarctions (heart attacks) in five to ten years. Insulin levels of 25 or above are diagnostic predictors of future heart problems.

A third cause of insulin resistance is obesity. Most people who are 30 pounds or more overweight have some degree of insulin resistance. Even many who are about eight to twelve pounds overweight, will exhibit several direct signs of insulin resistance. Weight loss of only fifteen pounds led to significant decreases in blood pressure in one study.

A fourth cause is overeating. This factor produces problems on its own, independent of the problems caused by overweight.

Physical inactivity also plays a significant part in insulin resistance. Regular exercise helps increase the utilization of sugar from the blood by the muscle cells, and assists in the appropriate use of insulin. Therefore, physical exercise is a good treatment for any feature of Syndrome X–overweight, high blood fats, diabetes, hypertension and heart disease.

Reduced blood flow to large muscle groups also appears to be a major cause of insulin resistance in most people with very high blood pressure. Possible causes for the reduced blood flow are little or no exercise, emotional tension, an inborn metabolic defect or reduced intake of magnesium and calcium. Both of these minerals relax the muscles and blood vessels. Chilled extremities, coffee or drug use will increase muscle tension. If muscles increase their uptake of blood when insulin goes up, blood pressure falls. Therefore, if people with hypertension do mild to moderate exercise after meals, they will increase blood flow to skeletal muscles and cause blood pressure to drop.[38]

Elevated insulin levels and insulin resistance can also occur from the quality of food in the diet. Humans are not careful to have good quality foods. Our passion for eating refined cereals, baked goods, and other carbohydrates is legendary in the western world. Thus, our typical diet of highly refined carbohydrates such as pastas from refined wheat, white rice, white flour, pastries, white bread, honey or sugar can lead to the very problems we are discussing, in many people.

Eating between meals is yet another form of incorrect eating leading to insulin resistance. The immediate results of incorrect eating, which cause a short period of elevated insulin levels, may take at least three days for the body to correct. So profound is the metabolic disorder in cells that the sugar and fat in one large chocolate bar can cause a weight gain of up to six pounds in fluid in the insulin resistant person.

Results of Insulin Resistance. Insulin resistance generates problems not only because of the other diseases associated with the genetic aspects, but also because of the extra insulin produced. An habitual excess of insulin in the blood stream for weeks or months has an effect on the body in several different ways as follows:

High blood pressure. Too much insulin in the

30

blood leads to hypertension by a complex mechanism.

Dyslipidemia. Lowering of HDL (good cholesterol) and raising of triglycerides and the harmful parts of the cholesterol fraction of the blood fats.

Damage to arteries. The longstanding elevation of insulin injures the heart and arteries in a still unknown process which results in atherosclerosis (hardening of the arteries). This process may work through liver disturbances.

The actual process of insulin resistance, high blood pressure and accompanying problems, is a pattern that includes the workings of several body mechanisms and systems. Excess insulin causes the kidneys to retain too much sodium and water with resultant increased tissue fluid and swelling of hands, feet, eyelids, etc. Excess insulin also increases the flow of sodium into the cell to toxic levels, which results in fluid retention and high blood pressure. Muscle cells are particularly responsive to changes in levels of sodium and potassium, leading to muscle cramps or headaches which may occur even before the blood pressure rises significantly.

The fluid environment outside the cells, the extracellular fluid, is partly made up of many kinds of ions, with sodium ions predominating. Inside the muscle cells, potassium predominates. When a muscle cell is stimulated it quickly becomes depolarized. For a split-second the electrical charge on the cell membrane reverses from negative to positive. Potassium rushes out of the cell and sodium rushes in. Sodium, calcium and magnesium trigger the cell to contract, or in the case of a nerve cell, to fire. While the potassium is out of the cell and the cell contains more sodium, a contraction takes place normally for a microsecond. This contraction, *when sustained in many cells simultaneously,* is what raises the blood pressure.

Normally, the sodium is ushered out of the cell, and potassium flows back into the cell as it retires into a resting state. But in insulin resistance, too many cells are going through this process without emptying the sodium completely, and then once again going into a period of rest. Because of this, tension on the muscles continues and the blood pressure stays up.

This causes a difficult predicament. The sodium molecule is much smaller than the potassium molecule and constantly diffuses into the cell through tiny pores. The functioning of the muscle and nerve cells is decreased when there is too much sodium diffusing in. Insulin resistance is one of the causes of this increased sodium flow into the cell. Also, the heart muscle does not function well when it is overburdened with too much sodium. A high salt diet loads excessive amounts of sodium into the extracellular fluid causing many problems with the sodium balance in the cells.

Interestingly, muscle and nerve cells are equipped with a "sodium pump." This "pump" works to dispose of the excess sodium in the blood, to keep blood levels normal. It is located in the membrane which surrounds the cell and normally acts somewhat like a conveyor belt to carry salt from the blood into the cells. Sodium is "trapped in its cogs" and conveyed across the cell membrane. Too much sodium in the blood overloads the "pump" and makes it malfunction.

Then the energy molecules, ATP, are not produced as much as are needed since the glucose of the body is not being oxidized as efficiently. An energy-deficient muscle cell becomes super-sensitive and spastic. This spasm in blood vessels will squeeze the blood and raise blood pressure.

Summary of Effects of Excess Insulin. A summary of excess insulin's effects on the body follows:
1. Excess insulin causes the kidneys to retain too much salt and water in the blood. This is why eating lots of Christmas holiday sweets, which boosts insulin levels, can cause sodium retention and the gaining of five to six pounds every week during the "sweets season." This process in-

32

creases the sodium concentration in blood vessel muscle cells. Then the blood vessels contract because they become overly sensitive to a hormone produced by the adrenals that elevates blood pressure.

2. High insulin levels retard the clearing of the blood of cholesterol, which then gets stuck to blood vessel linings. This factor increases the risk of coronary artery disease and hypertension. [41]

3. Excess insulin causes cramps and headaches.

4. Tension or prolonged contraction of skeletal muscle cells causes the blood pressure to go up. Skeletal muscle has been implicated as the major site of insulin resistance. [39] Exercise is the remedy of choice.

5. This tension or prolonged contraction will produce abnormal function of the heart muscle because of too much sodium in the cells.

6. Smooth muscle in blood vessel walls increases in size and strength. This increased size of the muscular walls increases the tension on the blood which pushes the blood pressure up.

7. Physical energy declines because ATP, the high energy molecule, does not receive adequate glucose to produce energy at full capacity.

8. When energy declines in a muscle cell, it responds by spasticity. The new tension on the muscles of the blood vessels causes the blood pressure to go up, further creating a vicious cycle.

9. Insulin stimulates the sympathetic nervous system which results in an elevation of stress hormones. A mother may notice that her children are disruptive and extremely overactive after eating sweets. When adults eat excessive sweets, the excess insulin produced can eventually cause their blood pressure to go up.

10. Both calcium and sodium increase inside muscle cells as insulin goes up in the blood. An excess of these minerals

also causes the muscles in the walls of the blood vessels
to be more sensitive and tight, which increases the blood
pressure.

11. Insulin is known to be a factor contributing to rapid body
growth in childhood. This growth factor causes not only
increased height and body fat, but also enlarged thickness
of blood vessel walls. In childhood, these conditions lay
the groundwork for hypertension in later life.

12. As insulin levels go up in the blood, there is interference
with the mechanism for keeping fibrinogen levels low.
Fibrinogen is part of the blood clotting process and can
increase the likelihood of hardening of the arteries with
resultant hypertension and coronary artery disease.[40] Most
likely, one of the reasons for increased heart attacks during holidays, is the increased intake of sweets which increases the potential to form clots within blood vessels.

34

other causes and effects of high blood pressure

There are several other causes of and effects from high blood pressure. High and low blood pressure can affect the **blood flow** to the hands and feet. It is assumed that blood flow to other organs is also affected, because the arteries act as a single organ. In severe hypertensives, the blood flow to the hands and feet is not as generous as in persons with normal blood pressure or only slightly elevated pressure.[69] The reduction in blood flow to the extremities may be a symptom of blood vessel disease or of chronic chilling.

There is an **increased viscosity** (the characteristic with which liquids flow; for example: honey has higher viscosity than water) in hypertensive subjects, both the increased plasma viscosity (liquid part of blood, not the cells) as well as increased hematocrits (proportion of red blood cells to plasma).[70] It appears that as the flow of blood inside the blood vessels becomes more like honey, the blood pressure climbs higher and higher. By a complex mechanism the increased pressure makes the blood flow even more like honey which causes the pressure to rise still further.

36   Factors which increase viscosity are dehydration, elevation of the number of red blood cells, increased blood cholesterol, high blood levels of salt, sugar, potassium, proteins, waste products and food substances being transported in the blood from the intestinal tract, especially foods having a high nutrient or calorie value. Check your lab values.

Chronic dehydration can also be a cause of high blood pressure. In his book, *Your Body's Many Cries For Water*, Dr. F. Batmanghelidj points out that high blood pressure and high blood cholesterol are two problems related to an always continuing deficiency of water in the body. The way to correct this chronic dehydration is to first reduce concentrated foods in the diet such as meat, milk, eggs, cheese, all refined foods (sugar, syrup, molasses, honey, white flour products, white rice, white starch and especially salt and salty foods), and foods high in free fats (margarine, butter, mayonnaise, fried foods, cooking fats, salad oils and nut butters). Increase water drinking to at least eight glasses per day. This can include caffeine-free herb teas. Do not use the decaffeinated teas or coffees because they contain other substances than caffeine which cause an elevation of blood pressure.

A **fast heart rate** has been associated with an increased incidence of getting hypertension, even in those people who begin with normal blood pressure. When a person who has been diagnosed with a higher than normal heart rate does not stay physically fit, his or her blood pressure is more likely to rise.

Hypertension also affects the **memory**. People suffering from even mild hypertension often lag behind those with normal blood pressure on several tests of memory and learning. It is not yet understood why this factor of memory is sensitive to elevated blood pressure; but somehow sustained high blood pressure may alter brain function and subtly interfere with mental activities, such as memory. Those who maintain an unhealthful lifestyle which results in hypertension, will have even more incentive to change their lifestyle once they realize the memory is also affected.[71] With hypertension, memory is slowed down but not lost, in contrast to Alzheimer's disease, in which the memory is actually lost.

For those who like to take warm baths and saunas, it is cheering to know that these hot treatments cause a slight reduction in blood pressure. But this reduction, unfortunately, appears to be temporary, and must be accompanied by lifestyle change to be long term.[72]

38

section two

lifestyle causes of hypertension

40

Case History

The following case shows how most people fail to make the connection between their close relatives and their own cases. It illustrates how it is necessary to study your family and then make adjustments in your life so that you have a good chance of avoiding the familial diseases which plagued your forebears and peers.

RL, a 58 year-old businessman from South Georgia wondered why he had developed high blood pressure. He was not much overweight and did not feel his life was particularly tense. He was a big man, six feet tall and 208 pounds. His mother, who was more than plump, had died of diabetes complicated by cancer of the large bowel and hypertension. But her lifestyle was very tense and although she was only 5'5" her weight was around 170. Even though his father was no more overweight than RL, he had died of a coronary heart attack at age 62. RL reasoned that his father was a smoker and since RL was not, he must therefore be at lower risk.

The businessman went to his doctor for a routine physical and his high blood pressure was discovered at 198/102; blood glucose 113, and cholesterol 325. Two years before his readings had been 132/82, 101, and 270; and four years before that, 120/76, 95, and 262. It was clear that his readings had been on the way up for many years but had taken a sudden jump. Now he needed a total change in lifestyle to avoid the same outcome as his parents.

He wanted to be treated without drugs and came to see us. He took a day of apple fasting, but could not make it through a day of water fasting. He did not want to become a vegetarian, and said he knew many people with heart disease who had not made major changes in their lifestyle--only weight reduction, stepped up exercise and a moderate reduction on margarine and red meat. He asked if we would treat him even if he continued to eat fish and white meat of poultry

42   as well as two eggs a week and some skim milk, as recommended by the American Heart Association. We saw fair changes in his blood pressure--150 to 160 for the systolic and 85 to 92 for the diastolic.

His weight steadily dropped to 182 then leveled off there. His cholesterol came down to 220 to 235 and stalled. After six months he began to lose ground. His weight crept up a few pounds, and his blood sugar for the first time showed a two-hours-after-meal reading above the laboratory normal of 115. His blood pressure bounced up to 180/95 and he returned to his original doctor who gave him medicines for his high sugar, his high cholesterol and his blood pressure.

Within 18 months he had had a bypass operation on his heart. Six months after the operation he developed angina on exertion. More medicines were added. Then he had an episode of bleeding from his bowel.

A polyp was removed from his colon which proved malignant. He tried to lose weight before bowel surgery and suddenly had to be rushed to the hospital with gallstones. Emergency surgery was followed by a stormy hospital course --an infection in his incision, another surgery to open and drain an abscess, a bout of pneumonia and then a severe heart attack.

We believe the diet of the American Heart Association is inadequate to protect people against a disastrous progression of heart and artery disease, eventually ending in a disabling or lethal event.

facts about stress and high blood pressure

Touching is generally associated with caring, compassion, sympathy and concern. Studies have been done showing that the soothing touch of another person produces a reduction in pulse rate and reduces blood pressure. From studies that have been done, it is logical to infer that touching will be associated with a generalized pattern of physiologic change (arousal reduction). Even monkeys respond with a decreased heart rate, to being stroked by humans.[49] Touching can be classed as another form of "laying on of hands." Even so, (as is illustrated in Chapter Thirteen in the story of Allie Mae Thomas) strong emotions can overcome compassionate touch.

Slow-stroke back massage has been shown to have a beneficial effect on both systolic and diastolic blood pressure.[50]

Perhaps one of the reasons relaxation and massage cause a fall in blood pressure is that they encourage the return of tissue fluid into the bloodstream. Relaxation does not give

44 everyone long-term benefits, but it usually brings the blood pressure down temporarily.[51]

A study done with a community of people who had never moved away from their home towns, had interesting findings. The study group maintained strong family and community ties throughout their entire lives. Although they ate the standard Western diet of meat, dairy, etc., their incidence of heart disease and high blood pressure was much lower than for the rest of the general population. This was attributed to the fact that they never had to experience the many trials, heartbreaks and insecurities of leaving family, friends, community and work. Neither did they ever have to encounter the difficulties involved in establishing new relationships or finding new work in an unfamiliar location. They maintained a lifelong, strong sense of security, which seems to have given them stable blood pressure readings and strong hearts.

Certain personality types have also been found to be more susceptible to high blood pressure than other types. The type A behavior personality is characterized by hostility and aggression, but is extremely organized, taking work home from the office, being a workaholic, speaking fast and even finishing sentences for other people.

These characteristics, accompanied by a corresponding intensification of the emotional state which causes blood vessels to constrict and blood flow to slow down, will often provoke a high incidence of hypertension and heart disease. It is possible that there could be also an associated mineral deficiency, such as magnesium, in these individuals to bring about their increased hypertension.[52] Rapid eating and emotional tension tend to cause magnesium to be poorly absorbed and utilized. A dose of Epsom salts, one-half to one teaspoon, taken twice daily, can be very helpful to restore magnesium balance. A more pleasant tasting magnesium salt is magnesium citrate, which is available in health food stores. But if rapid eating is a factor in hypertension, keep in mind that eating slowly has many other benefits. By taking time to eat, there will be fewer peptic ulcers, less digestive burdens on the pancreas and a lower rate of fermentation during digestion.

Other Types of Stress. It was discovered 50 years ago that the stress of overeating aggravates high blood pressure, completely apart from the excess salt or sodium taken in by overeating.[53] It is now recognized that the increased insulin required during the digestion of a large amount of food is part of the increased stress on the body (see Chapter Three on insulin resistance).

Another illustration of how stress increases blood pressure is shown by the rural South Africans. When they move from their country environment to the city, the ratio rises between the sodium they eat in their food, and the sodium they put out in urine. Their blood pressure also rises significantly.[54] In South African rural areas, a very natural lifestyle is followed. The people are not overweight. But the large cities with their noise, bustle, artificial lifestyles and rich, fast food diets, combine to take their toll on the health of the once robust, rural South African, now overweight, hypertensive and often nervous, anxious or depressed. No jails are necessary in the rural areas and the people are peace loving.

In a book entitled *Testimonies for the Church* (Volume 1:618), a Christian church leader once made the following statement:

"The abuses of the stomach by the gratification of appetite are the fruitful source of most church trials. [Certainly, the experience of the South Africans supports this.]

"Those who eat and work intemperately and irrationally, talk and act irrationally. An intemperate man cannot be a patient man. It is not necessary to drink alcoholic liquors in order to be intemperate. The sin of intemperate eating, eating too frequently, too much and of rich, unwholesome food, destroys the healthy action of the digestive organs, affects

46   *the brain and perverts the judgment, preventing rational, calm, healthy thinking and acting."* And this is the cause of many family, office and school trials!

"Therefore, in order for the people of God to be earnestly waiting in an acceptable state with Him, where they can glorify Him in their bodies and in their spirits which are His, they must with interest and zeal deny gratification of their unhealthful appetites, and exercise temperance in all things. Then may they comprehend the truth in its beauty and clearness, and carry it out in their lives, and by a judicious, wise, straightforward course give the enemies of our faith no occasion to reproach the cause of truth. God requires all who believe the truth to make special, persevering efforts to place themselves in the best possible condition of bodily health, for life is a solemn and important work.

"Health of body and mind is required for this work: it is as essential to a healthy religious experience, to advancement in the Christian life and progress in holiness, as is the hand or foot to the human body. God requires His people to cleanse themselves from all filthiness of the flesh and spirit, perfecting holiness in the fear of the Lord. All those who are indifferent and excuse themselves from this work, waiting for the Lord to do for them that which he requires them to do for themselves, will find that their lives exhibit a weakness which they would not reveal if only they had learned moderation in all things--total abstinence from things hurtful and the temperate use of all things beneficial."

The Effect of Conversation on Blood Pressure   Certain everyday activities, such as conversing with one another, which we would never suspect of having an impact on our blood pressure, actually have more of an effect than we imagine. Conversation, even when it is quiet and casual, can cause an increase in blood pressure and cardiac output equivalent to that of moderate exercise. [55] It is for this reason that the conventional techniques used in the measuring of blood pres-

47

sure using the stethoscope and a blood pressure cuff, require silence during the evaluation. Conversation can rapidly increase systolic and diastolic pressures, in some situations greater than 20%, within 30 seconds of initiating speech. More rapid speech and an increased output of words has been associated with higher blood pressure levels.[56]

The Effect of Noise on Blood Pressure. Studies show that noise can impair the proper functioning of the cardiovascular system and may trigger high blood pressure.[57] The mean blood pressures in subjects with noise-induced loss of hearing were significantly higher than those found in subjects with normal hearing acuity.[58]

To test the effects of noise on blood pressure, monkeys were inundated for three weeks straight with the sounds of traffic, TV, telephones and alarm clocks. The monkeys' blood pressures rose by 43%.[59] Our contemporary city living with the constant bombardment and clamor of radio, TV, stereos, tape players, sirens and street noises encourage not only hearing loss but elevation of blood pressure.

Temperature and Blood Pressure. Cold and heat have quite a striking influence on the blood pressure in many individuals. The response to the "cold pressor test" has shown that in many people, there is a distinct response in blood pressure to chilling of even one extremity. Even cold weather tends to bring a higher overall blood pressure reading than hot weather. Blood pressure readings begin to go up in November and stay up until April. In May,

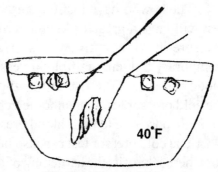

40°F

The Cold Pressor Test

48   they start to go down again and reach their lowest point in September. [60]

The cold pressor test is based on the fact that in response to a cold stimulus, the arterial blood pressure goes up. A normal person increases diastolic by about 5mm and systolic by 15-20mm. A hypo-reactor has less than the normal increases and a hyper-reactor has greater than normal increases.

The test is basically simple. The first thing the patient must do is to rest in a quiet room, either sitting or lying down, for 15 minutes to one hour. Then a blood pressure cuff is applied to one arm and a basal pressure reading taken. Leave the blood pressure cuff on the arm. The free hand, up to just above the wrist, is then immersed in cold water at 40-59 degrees for five minutes. Blood pressure readings must be taken every minute for the five minutes. Write down each reading and compare with the first, resting level. If the highest reading does not go up more than 5/2, (that is, 5 on the systolic reading and 2 on the diastolic reading) the person is a hyporeactor, or one who does not react as rapidly as expected; about 15/5 is normal; over 20/15, the person is at risk for cardiovascular disease within the next 10 years; more than 50/20, the risk is acute. [61]

Those who have a strong response to the cold pressor test will have a greater likelihood of developing high blood pressure in the next five years. Transient vasoconstriction (temporary tightening of blood vessels) precedes the rise in blood pressure. The rise in blood pressure associated with the cold pressor test is an inherited characteristic and appears to predispose one to high blood pressure. [62]

The cold pressor test can also be used as a screening test for atherosclerosis, the hardening of the arteries resulting usually from a very damaging lifestyle. Hypertensive patients have been found with testing to have an accelerated rate of developing atherosclerosis.[63]

In 641 patients with atherosclerosis, if atherosclerosis

existed alone or in combination with the high blood pressure, there was a greater reaction to the test than in normal controls.[64]

We have all heard of the "Polar Bear Clubs," made up of individuals who swim in ice cold waters in winter. These swimmers claim to be unusually strong because they have the fortitude to endure the icy waters. They also claim that the cold water has a beneficial effect on their health. But in tests done on a group of 28 people who regularly "enjoyed" swimming in near freezing waters, their blood pressures revealed they had an unusually high degree of hypertension. One had 180/105 and three had a diastolic value of 95 and above. Ideal values run below 120/80. Systolic blood pressure increased significantly while the subjects were waiting undressed in the cold air in a cabin by the pond. Neither immersion nor swimming in the ice cold water caused further increase in the systolic pressure.[65] Perhaps the so-called "white coat hypertension" may be due in part to some degree of chilling from being undressed except for a very thin examination gown.

These observations underscore the importance of proper clothing of the extremities. Check your clothing. The skin on the back of the upper arms should be as warm as the forehead. So should other key areas: the side of the thigh, the ankle and the top of the foot. Put on more clothing if necessary!

Swimming in ice cold waters is accompanied by a fair amount of shivering. But it can take a far less dramatic stimulus than a swim in frigid waters, to start shivering. Being out in the rain with improper clothing, sitting near a draft or getting out of a warm shower and stepping into a cold room, can all result in shivering. When you begin to shiver, it is an indication that the body temperature has fallen and the blood pressure has risen. The intensity of shivering rises and falls in step with the highs and lows of the blood pressure.[66]

50

Other blood pressure tests using cold water have been devised. In one test, 42 healthy, young adults were subjected to immersion in cold water and responded by an immediate and marked elevation of the arterial pressure. Over 94% of the subjects reached maximum systolic elevation between 40 and 70 seconds after immersion. About 96% of the group reached their maximum diastolic elevation within 30 seconds. The average systolic elevation was 22.6 mm and the average diastolic elevation was 16.3 mm.[67]

Blood pressure can be raised by something as simple as drinking three glasses of icy beverage. The volume of liquid is as important as the temperature. If about three ice-cold glasses of liquid were drunk, the systolic pressure in test subjects generally increased by 10 mm.[68]

Even if a custom is widely accepted, it can be unhealthful. The practice of dressing as scantily as is feasible is a practice hazardous to the blood pressure. Habitual chilling of the extremities not only increases the risk of developing hypertension, but also reduces the effectiveness of the immune system. It has been shown that more women in cold climates tend to have breast cancer than women in warm climates. This may be due in part to habitual chilling of the extremities. With high blood pressure, as with any other illness, emotional factors are involved. Stress, compulsive excitement and hilarious laughter, and those unresolved troublesome situations, unhappiness, depression or anxiety are several of the emotional states that contribute to high blood pressure.

Suppressing or hiding these problems can mean a higher risk of heart disease. Studies have shown that people who hide psychological distress, from themselves and others, may show an overreaction of the cardiovascular system to stress, which can lead to a higher risk of heart disease, high blood pressure and irregular and/or fast heartbeat. These early malfunctions can also be the forerunners to heart attacks. Lack of social support, hostility and work-related stresses also contribute to the overall stress on the blood pressure and heart.[43] A good relationship with our Heavenly Father will relieve this kind of risk of disease.

When sudden stresses or trials beset a person, the blood pressure immediately goes up, at least to a small degree. Life's little or big changes which are perceived to be negative will also cause the blood pressure to go up in people who are susceptible to hypertension.[44] The increased pressure in the blood vessels causes a rapid shift of water out of the bloodstream into the tissues. The body then reacts with metabolic stress (added to psychological stress) which can cause the blood pressure to remain high in the susceptible person. [45]

At times our lives are filled with events and feelings that are so intense, we cannot deal with them alone. Hostility, or life events that evoke a hostile response, are associated with greater diastolic blood pressure.[46]

Then it is time to select a counselor to help sort out confusing circumstances and emotions, and assist in the process of putting life into a proper perspective. Godly Christian counselors are available, who will lead clients to depend on Christ for help in straightening out hurting hearts. Don't hesitate to call on a trained, Bible-based counselor if you feel you need assistance. Seventh-day Adventist churches have pastors and others experienced in such work. In the next chapter are suggestions to help you cope with your emotions in a healthful and heart-preserving manner.

52

what to do for emotional and psychological factors

Perhaps the most delicate work we ever do is that of changing the basic stresses of life, of deciding what God's will is for the life, and then being consistent in instituting the changes needed. In this chapter we give suggestions that, if faithfully followed, will result in reducing your stress level.

Treatment of Emotional and Psychological Factors.

1. *Confront each problem in your life.* Acknowledge the fact that your problems cause you discomfort, even though you may not consciously "feel" any uneasiness. Hiding psychological troubles may come with a price tag. Your body may register your discomfort in the form of high blood pressure or some other problem, even if your conscious mind doesn't want to admit to difficulties. In one study it was discovered that people with hidden psychological distress, hidden from themselves as well as from others, showed an

54

unusual jump in heartbeat and blood pressure when doing stressful tasks. [47, 48]

Examine all your problems carefully, both those that are yours alone and those that include your closest associates. Recognize that it is part of the human condition to have problems; if you belong to the human race, you will have problems. Too often our society dictates that it is not acceptable to have problems, but don't believe this. Those who are the loudest proponents of this error are most likely the ones with the biggest problems.

Become a person of prayer. Study the Bible with its promises of close daily interaction of heavenly beings in the affairs of men. We need not lack wisdom. God is gracious and loving and wants you to be well and happy. Ask for His help in searching your heart. Pray for the people with whom you want to improve your communication and relationship and ask God to help you--with family, friends, co-workers, and even daily acquaintances.

Observe your emotions and your usual way of life. Are you frequently angry? Do you have hidden angers you need to recognize and deal with? Do many things in life cause you frustration? Do you harbor resentments? Do you push yourself way beyond your limits? Do you try to control other people? These types of emotions and habits can cause elevation in blood pressure.

Accept the fact that you will have to make some changes in your life, both emotional and physical, if you want to improve your health. You may have to do unfamiliar things and break out of self-defeating behavior patterns. But all of these changes become easier as you pray for divine assistance and apply every known health principle.

2. *Make exercise a daily part of your schedule.* While exercising, meditate on the goodness of God and the natural world He has made. **Never rehearse your problems**. Al-

though we are unworthy, He has offered us salvation from disease as well as salvation from sin. Interestingly, the word salvation comes from the same root word as "salve."

3. *Be regular in all your daily habits.* A certain amount of peace comes merely from having a schedule and following it as closely as possible with all routine events such as meals, sleep, exercise, study, prayer and worship.

4. *Prayer is the breath of the soul.* Fresh prayer throughout the day, on every topic which comes to mind, keeps the soul in communion with our Heavenly Father and helps us walk with God as Enoch did. Calmness floods the soul and a joy fills the heart with singing. Cultivate a cheerful demeanor. Be thankful in all things, even when they may seem like disasters. Even grieving a loss can bring joy, but not without Christ. Sorrow does not need to be associated with depression, but can be associated with joy in Christ.

Thomas Edison was in his 60's when his workshop and warehouse went up in smoke. When his son saw his father watching the blaze, his heart broke in sympathy for the older man. He knew that much of his life's work, equipment and plant, worth over $500,000--quite a lot in those days--was going up in smoke. But Thomas Edison said, "Son, there is value even in a destructive fire. All our mistakes are burned up." Three weeks later Edison developed the world's first wireless radio. Had he yielded to the emotions his son expected him to have he might never have made this contribution to the world.

5. *Organize your home life* and make changes where necessary. A neat and orderly home promotes household happiness. Following are several ways to develop orderliness in the home:

> *Do not neglect family government.* Meet together daily for singing, worship, prayer and study. Mother and Father should be the kindly managers of the home. Children are the subjects of their

administration.

Teach respect for one another and for the principles of the Bible. Don't allow teasing or belittling, which weaken the emotions and the spirit.
Maintain the most healthful diet. For hypertension, heart disease, diabetes and overweight the
most healthful diet is a total vegetarian diet; no
meat, milk, eggs or cheese. Begin to approach
this diet as a lifestyle change, not just a temporary measure. You have already proven your old
lifestyle to lead to hypertension and probably
other disabling diseases. Use a varied diet of
fruits, vegetables, whole grains, nuts and seeds.
In most cases free fats--margarine, butter, fried
foods, cooking fats, salad oils and nut butters--
should be eliminated. Learn mouth-watering substitutes. See Chapter Fourteen for some additional
information.

6. *Avoid noise and confusion of all kinds.* This includes loud
music, especially of the rock or rap variety. Television can
be a real source of very significant stresses and confusion.
On a radio talk show in the mid-nineties, a researcher indicated that the average American adult will spend 14 years
watching TV during a lifetime. That represents a lot of
stress bombardment!

7. *Follow Bible instruction.* The Bible instructs us that we
may treat illness by calling the elders of the church together
for prayer and anointing.

*"Is any among you afflicted? Let him pray....Is
any sick among you? Let him call for the elders of
the church; and let them pray over him, anointing him
with oil in the name of the Lord: and the prayer of
faith shall save the sick, and the Lord shall raise him
up; and if he have committed sins, they shall be for-
given him. Confess your faults one to another, and*

pray one for another, that ye may be healed. The effectual fervent prayer of a righteous man availeth much." James 5:13-16 The Lord in Heaven is enabled to do for us that which He cannot do in the great plan of salvation if we do not thus pray.

Case History

The following case report is that of a dear lady who was never willing to get a grip on her life until after she had a devastating stroke which left her with a permanent limp and a weak left hand. How much better for her changes to come before the stroke than after.

IHM, a pleasant, 63 year old school teacher from north Alabama, was a frequent patient in our lifestyle center, and a regular visitor on campus, as her daughter was a staff member of Uchee Pines Institute. She always enjoyed being here, saying that if she could live here permanently she could lose the 40 pounds she needed, get her blood pressure and diabetes under control, and perhaps feel better with her arthritis. Her blood pressure hovered around 200/98 and her blood sugar readings went as high as 350. She refused to take insulin or medicines of any kind.

When she had finished a patient session, she would have lost eight or ten pounds, would get in good enough physical condition by the end of the three weeks to walk two to four miles each day, and would say, "I am a new woman."

When anyone from our institute visited her, they found ice cream in her freezer, cake in the refrigerator, chocolate chip cookies on the counter, and used napkins from the local Dairy Queen. She loved chips and anything else salty, and ignored her blood pressure. One time I saw some of these items in her car trunk when I helped her put her bags in the car. "What are these doing in your car?" She explained she had been having a struggle with her appetite before she came.

68   *I asked, "Would you like me to dispose of them for you?"
She said she would give them to her son's children as soon as
she got home. "Are you sure you can trust your appetite
now? You know you always come here having gained back
all the weight you lost the last time. Your blood pressure and
diabetes are not to be trifled with; they can be very destruc-
tive." She closed her trunk with a big smile and was gone,
waving cheerfully.*

*That was the last time I saw her before her stroke. Two
months later her son called me in tears to say his mother had
suffered a very devastating stroke and was paralyzed on the
left side. She was unconscious and unable to swallow. Her
improvement was slow, but after she was using a walker she
came to stay a few weeks with her daughter. From then until
she died six years later she lived a model lifestyle. If anyone
offered her a dessert, she quietly refused. Her weight came
down to 125 pounds and her blood pressure was never over
118/78. Even though she now had all her health measure-
ments in order, this was the end of her usefulness and much
of her joy in living. Most of the rest of her life was spent
merely taking care of herself, with generous help from relatives and friends.*

diet and blood pressure

While we are still only beginning to understand the role of diet in controlling body processes, much has been learned, and more information is constantly being discovered. As we noted in the first part of this book, in spite of what many older physicians still believe, what we eat has a great deal to do with blood pressure. If we are in the habit of eating meats and dairy products, overeating, using extra salt in our cooking and at the table and eating in fast-food restaurants, we will greatly increase our risk of high blood pressure.

If what we eat raises blood pressure, it makes sense to stop eating the things that are harmful. With some study and experimentation with cookbooks, you can actually enjoy eating more of those foods which are beneficial. In time you will not recognize the clamor of the appetite which has been a source of such trouble. Remembering some of the problems brought on by continuing in an unhealthful lifestyle will nerve you to press forward until you have firmly established the new habits. Sometimes two or three years are required to galvanize the new habits into a comfortable, automatic and permanent lifestyle, requiring no special thought or provision.

60   This may mean forsaking your favorite foods. But as you learn to eat differently, you will find new favorites, and what at first seemed like an indescribable loss, is transformed into an enthusiasm for more healthful foods. Even people who love salt and have strong food preferences which they forcefully defend, find that when they give the new eating program a three-week trial, a new set of food preferences gradually develops along with an easing of the grip of old food cravings. You will discover that eating what you know will hurt you is no longer something you want to do, or are driven to do. The improvement in sense of well-being is encouragement enough to stick to the beneficial changes. It is important, that when advances are made in changing the appetite, no ground should be lost by even a single regression into old habits. It is no favor to yourself to indulge appetite. *Weeks of guilt and remorse over failure can sometimes be the result of even one little indulgence.*

Even though changing the way we are accustomed to eating sounds like a burdensome chore, it can be made into an exciting adventure; a journey onto a path of new culinary delights. We have to learn how to take familiar staple foods, like whole grains and fresh vegetables, off the shelves and put them into the cooking pots. The fine art of seasoning will have to be practiced. Delve into cookbooks which explain how to prepare fresh foods and make them into delectable meals. Ask longtime vegetarians how they season vegetables, salads, soups, etc. At first it may be a terrible struggle to make so many changes. But after a few weeks of practice, you will be able to easily cook delicious, healthful meals as well as save time and money.

You will find as you begin to eat differently, your tastes change. Foods that once appealed to you—the high-fat, high-salt foods—no longer seem as palatable. Instead of grabbing a bite at a fast-food restaurant, you will be more eager to get home to "Grade A" food your body requires to function at its best. When you no longer have high blood pressure you will look with pleasure on your new lifestyle. Added benefits include lowered risk for all the major lifestyle diseases we face today, such as cancer, heart disease, overweight, diabetes, arthritis and others.

Family and friends can be the biggest encouragements or the stubbornest obstacles to your new eating program. If they do not believe that changing the way you eat will make a difference in your health, you have to firmly continue with your new diet, no matter what they may say. Sometimes, entire families join in the new diet while other families refuse. Be determined, and pray that your family will make no belittling or humorous remarks about your efforts to become well. Maintain a cheerful attitude. Never discuss food changes when you and your family are hungry! Wait until you have all eaten a full meal. Your family will be more willing to accept changes when their stomachs are full.

Learning new habits, like new eating habits that involve a large portion of your life, takes time and much patience. But the rewards of the struggle are far greater than expected, especially in terms of prolonging your youth and usefulness, and the avoidance of higher risk of living with a crippling complication of high blood pressure.

Lifestyle changes of reduction in weight and dietary sodium, eliminating alcoholic beverage intake, and increase in physical activity should be the first line of approach to the treatment of hypertension. [135]

Salt, fat, sugar and other nutrients

Salt. Americans eat far too much salt (sodium chloride). Americans also eat far too much food. Since most foods contain some sodium naturally, it is not essential for good nutrition for most people to add any salt to food during cooking or

62 at the table. Lowering the intake of salt might require some adjustments of habits. But it is of great benefit for the prevention or treatment of elevated blood pressure in susceptible people.

Sodium to a large degree controls the quantity of water in the blood volume, and the quantity of lymph fluid held in the tissues between the cells.

The volume of blood is regulated very precisely by the kidneys over a 24 hour period. All the salt ingested the previous day will be excreted in the urine except for that which we have put out in sweat, milk, blood loss, or fluid lost by mouth droplets or in nasal secretions. The kidneys regulate exactly how much sodium must be eliminated to maintain proper blood volume, which is essential for life.

We take in a lot of sodium from table salt, baking powder, soft drinks, mineral waters and foods. Sodium, or table salt sensitivity is now being experienced by many people, especially seen within certain families. These people are more likely to get hypertension. For most people, removing some of the salt from their food results in a decrease in blood pressure. For some there is no effect. And for an occasional person there is an actual increase in blood pressure from restricting salt intake.[73] Test your blood pressure both before and after salt restriction to determine the kind of person you are.

The importance of eating more fresh fruits and vegetables and less food in general cannot be overemphasized for most hypertensives. Fruits especially are very low in salt, and generally taste better without salt than any other class of food. Blood pressure diets should emphasize fruits as tasty and healthful. Furthermore, eating a smaller quantity of food reduces the total quantity of salt since even natural foods contain some salt. Training the appetite to accept less food will generally have a noticeably beneficial effect on the blood pressure.

When we eat too much salt, the body cannot handle the excess properly. In Northern Japan and Evans County, Georgia, the two places where the inhabitants have the highest salt consumption in the world, a high salt intake has been associated with a high death rate from strokes. Too much sodium in the diet causes salt to be processed in the body in an abnormal manner, such as the way the salt is transported across cell membranes. The sodium pump which transports sodium across cell membranes will not work properly in the presence of excess salt in the diet. It has been shown that white and red blood cells of hypertensive patients, have abnormal sodium transport mechanisms apparently since birth.[74, 75]

As for the salt substitutes, it is best that they not be used. These substitutes tend to cause problems for the body in other ways. While sodium chloride, regular table salt or sea salt, may be harmful in overdosage in one way, other salts such as lithium chloride or potassium chloride are both harmful in overdosage in other ways.[76]

Tips to Reduce Sodium Intake Steps to take to reduce salt in the diet begin in the grocery store. The following suggestions for low-salt shopping can also be used as a preventive measure by those who are not now suffering with high blood pressure.

1. *When shopping, whenever possible select fresh foods* from the produce section rather than processed foods. Processed foods are foods in boxes, cans, bottles, etc. There are many recipes of delicious food which are good for hypertensives, using fresh foods in our cookbook, *Eat For Strength*. When you must buy something processed, choose no-salt products. Mix your own salad dressings with blended tomatoes, garlic and lemon juice and leave the oil, salt and vinegar off your table. See *Eat for Strength Oil-Free Edition*.[77]

2. *Prepare your own meals* whenever possible, using only the freshest ingredients. Learn how to select or grow

64

herbs such as basil, dill, parsley, marjoram, etc., to make your dishes tasty while leaving the salt out of your recipes. There are many different no-salt seasonings available in the market, suitable for table use, which are excellent salt replacements and which will add a delicious flavor to your meals. Investigate these.

3. *Become a label reader.* When you must choose processed food, make sure you read the ingredients. If you find salt listed, leave that food on the shelf. Products like soy sauce, tomato juice, monosodium glutamate, milk--especially nonfat milk--olives and bacon-like bits have large amounts of hidden salt. If it is a product such as olives or canned garbanzo beans, part of the salt can be rinsed off with water. Some of the nutrients will be lost with the rinsing, but this will not be a nutritional problem, as long as you do not eat prepared foods often.

There are even foods which are not usually considered salty but are known to contain considerable quantities of salt. Dark *Karo* syrup, for example, contains an unexpected listing of salt.[78] Get in the habit of reading all labels!

Some foods which we expect to have only a small amount of salt are actually loaded with salt, like *Campbell*'s tomato juice. Only six ounces (one quarter less than a full glass) contains 570 milligrams of sodium. That is more than half the daily allotment for a hypertensive patient!

4. *Certain foods have a naturally high content of sodium,* while other foods have a low content. Below is a partial listing of **high-sodium foods**:
   - Beverages called "sodas"
   - Breads raised with baking powder (often contain sodium bicarbonate)
   - Chips
   - Cheese
   - Commercially prepared sauces

•Milk (natural salt from the cow!)
•Tomato products (soup, juice, sauces, and vending machine items)
Now, for some of the naturally **low-sodium foods**:
•Fruits (all!)
•Homemade foods, no salt added
•Nuts and seeds, unsalted
•Pasta, home cooked, unsalted
•Rice, cooked with no salt
Learn to read the nutrition information on packages.

5. *Many drugs have large quantities of sodium.* An example is penicillin. Zantac has no salt in the tablets, but the effervescent tablets contain 370 milligrams! Many antacids, commonly taken for indigestion, were formerly high in sodium. However, manufacturers became aware that people were avoiding their product because of the sodium content. Now, most antacids will give 2.5 milligrams or less of salt per dose. But if one is taking them at the maximum allowable dosage (24 teaspoons in 24 hours), it would be possible to take in up to 60 milligrams from this source alone. There are other drawbacks to antacids and they are best completely avoided. If you are eating properly, indigestion will rarely occur and there will be no need to take antacids. The following is a list of antacids:

Table For Antacids

Tums, suspension and tablets
Milk of Magnesia
ALTERNAGEL Liquid
Alu-Cap Capsules and Alu-Tab Tablets
Amphojel Tablets
Basaljel Capsules
Maalox
Mylanta
Riopan

66   When the body is forced to deal with too much salt, its organs become overworked trying to process the excess. If the kidneys cannot get rid of the surplus, the body will retain water to keep the salt diluted. The resulting increase in volume of blood keeps the amount of blood the heart pumps high, resulting in its beating forcefully.[79] This raises the blood pressure. The kidneys are damaged by too much salt and begin to develop injuries in their microscopic structure. The chemical products made by the kidney are then altered. One of these chemicals causes the blood vessels to contract, pushing the blood pressure up. The elevated pressure damages the blood vessels over an extended period of time and fat begins to deposit inside the damaged areas of the vessel walls. This leads to hardening of the arteries which eventually causes heart attacks or strokes.

In addition to salt restriction, the initial recovery program of a person with high blood pressure should include quitting smoking, stopping alcohol consumption, beginning regular daily aerobic exercise, a vegan vegetarian diet to insure adequate intake of potassium, magnesium and calcium, and the elimination of saturated fats and cholesterol.[80]

Fats. Fats, as well as salt, have been found to have a negative influence on persons who have problems with blood pressure. Fat consumption has been shown in numerous studies to be associated with a rise in blood pressure. This has been shown in dogs,[81] humans, [82, 83] and in rabbits.[84] Americans commonly eat diets which include too many meats and dairy products; both are excessively rich in fat. Our bodies cannot continuously handle this overload of fat without eventually developing a diseased condition.

In specialized feeding studies done with rats, it was found that a diet high in both fat and salt caused the highest elevation of blood pressure, more than fat or salt alone.[85] This information persuades us to reflect on our current eating habits, such as commercially baked, canned and junk foods, to see where we can make changes and adjustments that will help us guard our health.

Free Fats May Cause Sticky Red Blood Cells.

Our Divine Designer placed an electrical charge on blood cells to keep them apart. Since similarly charged bodies repel each other, red blood cells with their charged skins, do not stick to each other unless the natural charge is neutralized.

Free fats (margarine, butter, mayonnaise, fried foods, cooking fats, salad oils and nut butters) in the blood neutralize the charge on red blood cell membranes, and promote clumping of red blood cells which reduces the free transport of oxygen. When oxygen falls, blood pressure goes up in an attempt to supply the shortage.

Sugar. Essential hypertension is very often related to the same genetic axis as diabetes. Many studies done with animals have found an association between excess consumption of sugars (sucrose, fructose and glucose) and elevated blood pressure.[86]

It is to the hypertensive patient's advantage to avoid sugar and all refined carbohydrates as much as possible, and maintain a similar type of program a diabetic uses. See Chapter Three on how blood pressure is related to other modern diseases such as diabetes.

As with the diabetic, a program of vigorous exercise, weight control, a totally vegetarian diet, a moderate or small amount of food and avoidance of refined food products, improves functioning of all the insulin receptors and greatly reduces hypertension.

It is difficult for the person with high blood pressure to understand that he or she has a metabolic problem involving the hormone system, but it is usually the case.

The principle hormones involved are insulin and adrenal hormones. (See our book, *Diabetes and The Hypoglycemic Syndrome.*) Some herbs that may help to stabilize the

68 hormone system are fenugreek, dandelion, aloe, blackberry, garlic, ginseng, goldenseal, raspberry and white willow.

Nutrients: Minerals

Minerals are nutrients found in certain foods. They help the body maintain an acid-base balance in the blood by moving in and out of the blood, bones and muscles as needed. Minerals are essential for nerve impulse transmission, muscle contraction, clotting of the blood, water balance and bone formation. They also regulate enzyme systems, give strength to certain structures (as calcium and zinc give to bone) and form parts of certain hormones, as iodine forms part of the thyroid hormone. Several minerals and other nutrients are important for maintaining blood pressure at normal levels. The following nutrients are also known to be important:

1. **Boron**. Boron is essential to properly build bones and muscles. This makes it important to the control of blood pressure. Furthermore, when the diet contains plenty of boron, there is a normalizing in blood levels of testosterone for both men and women. Don't think, however, that you can accomplish proper hormone levels or get larger muscles from taking a supplement from a bottle, as supplementing does not further increase testosterone or promote muscle growth. [131] Food sources include legumes (beans and peas) and certain fruit--apples, pears, grapes and their juices.

2. **Iron**. This mineral is a major part of hemoglobin. Hemoglobin is the blood protein which carries oxygen. Foods high in iron include green leafy vegetables, beans, prunes, dried apricots, raisins, grapes, apples, nuts and whole grains. If the iron level is too high in the blood, the blood pressure may rise. The hemoglobin and serum iron should be maintained on the low side of normal for the best functioning of the cardiovascular system, the immune system and the blood cell system. For women the ideal hemoglobin level

should be between 10.5-12.5, and for men between 12-14. Serum iron, ideally, should probably be kept between 30-80. If your levels are too high, you may be helped by donating blood regularly to the Red Cross. Donate as frequently as allowed until your levels are lowered to the ideal. You are not necessarily sick because your iron levels are high, any more than if your body weight is high. Do not say to the person interviewing you that you have a condition for which you need to give blood, or you will be considered a therapeutic donor and will require a doctor's order and will have to pay. You should qualify as a donor if you have no other condition.

3. *Magnesium*. One of its major purposes involves the nutrition and function of muscle cells and health of the nerves. It may control growth and help regulate the workings of all body functions. Since insulin can enhance transport of magnesium into cells, people with a genetic background of diabetes or insulin resistance usually develop a deficiency of magnesium. [87]

Many systems in the body depend on magnesium in order to function. Magnesium interacts with other minerals and some trace elements and nutrients--potassium, calcium, sodium and zinc, and is essential to the nutrition of cardiac muscle cells. Some good researchers believe the reason we are hearing so much about mitral valve prolapse, is because of a general deficiency of magnesium in Western diets which results in chronic magnesium deficiency in cardiac muscle. Magnesium deficiency has been associated with a number of diseases, including high blood pressure, heart rhythm disturbances, heart attacks and diabetes. It is also possible that chronic magnesium depletion is responsible for metabolic bone diseases such as osteoporosis. [88]

Chlorine encourages magnesium deficiency by decreasing absorption and increasing excretion. It does the

70

same thing for calcium and phosphorus. Therefore, we recommend to hypertensives that they not use water to which chlorine has been added.[89]

A study of 30,681 men aged 40–75 without hypertension or other known disease revealed that as the intake of magnesium went up in the diet, blood pressures went down; as fiber went up, blood pressures went down.

The same was discovered for potassium and calcium. The most favorable diet to provide these nutrients is one high in fruits, vegetables, whole grains, legumes, nuts and seeds.[90]

Certain common practices also cause a loss of magnesium in the urine. Drinking soft drinks which contain quantities of phosphates, salt and sugar; the use of tobacco, and alcohol have all been associated with magnesium loss. The use of diuretics causes a significant loss of magnesium, in addition to sodium and potassium.

Taking mineral supplements is not always a wise idea in normal people, as major

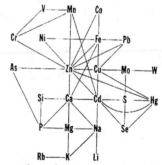

Interactions of Micronutrients (Minerals)

If one mineral goes up, minerals on a line with it go down.

imbalances in the nutrient economy of the body may occur. Note the diagram showing the relationship of minerals with each other. If one mineral is taken in overdose, minerals having a dependancy on that mineral may get thrown off balance. For example, if iron is taken as a supplement, cobalt, calcium and zinc may become imbalanced. It is best to be fairly certain of a deficiency, or aim at a specific disease as a trial, before embarking on a long term course of mineral supplementation. Persons with hypertension are justified in taking a trial course of a couple of months of a magnesium supplement.

Foods high in magnesium include bananas, whole grains, dry beans, nuts, peanut butter and dark green, leafy vegetables.

4. *Potassium*. Potassium acts as a major regulator of the blood pressure. Increased potassium in the diet may be what accounts for the low incidence of hypertension in vegetarians.[91] Foods high in potassium are potatoes, kidney beans, peas, bananas, oranges and dried fruits which can actually decrease blood pressure by 5-15 points.[92]

5. *Calcium*. Calcium also helps to lower blood pressure. Foods high in calcium are dry beans and peas, whole grains, greens, figs, sesame seeds and broccoli. Milk is not a good source of calcium for the hypertensive because of its high fat, high salt and high phosphate content. Foods high in phosphate (red meats, dairy cheeses, soft drinks and baking powder) cause a loss of calcium because of the seesaw relationship these two nutrients have.

A study done with 6,634 men and women at the University of Southern California School of Medicine in Los Angeles, beginning in 1971 and ending in 1984, revealed that the use of foods very high in calcium (sufficient to supply 1000 milligrams per day) can lower high blood pressure by an average of 12%. No hypertensives were in the group at the start. Those who drank alcohol on a daily basis got no benefit from calcium intake. Those under age 40 were benefited even more: a 25% reduction in blood pressure from foods supplying 1000 milligrams of calcium per day.[93]

6. *Certain minerals* are unfortunately also related to an elevation in blood pressure. High barium levels in public drinking water have been discovered to increase blood pressure.[94]

Nutrients: Amines, Vitamins and Their Sources

72

1. *Myoinositol,* a nutrient found abundantly in a vegetarian diet, especially cantaloupe, citrus and legumes, is deficient in those who are insulin-resistant.[95] See Chapter Three on insulin resistance. This nutrient helps reduce the ill effects of insulin resistance, a factor in hypertension. See a more complete listing in Appendix.

2. *Certain commercial nutrient supplements* such as calcium and vitamin C, when taken in large doses can raise blood pressure.[96] But calcium also has a diuretic effect. In many studies blood pressure actually decreased by giving calcium carbonate. Depending on the circumstances and the dosage, calcium can raise or lower blood pressure.[97] Study your own reaction to calcium and vitamin C supplements if you take them.

3. *Since the entire subject* of treatment with mineral and vitamin supplements is a controversial topic, caution is recommended to avoid injury from overdoses of supplements.

4. *Amines,* building blocks for proteins which contain nitrogen, are found in all natural foods. They have varying effects on blood pressure. Carl Pfeiffer, M.D., found one amine, histamine, to cause the blood pressure to rise. Histamine is found in small amounts in certain vegetables such as spinach and eggplant. It is also found in much larger amounts (along with tyramine), in cheeses, especially Parmesan, blue and Roquefort, and in red wines like Chianti and Burgundy.[98]

5. *Taurine,* an amino acid-like nutrient, found in mother's milk (but not in cow's milk), as well as in some food sources, will lower blood pressure.[99, 100] Interestingly, it has both a developing and a regenerative effect on nerve tissue. Babies raised on mother's milk instead of cow's milk have an average measurable IQ elevation of five points over babies raised on cow's milk. Legumes, nuts and seeds are also good sources. (See Appendix for full listing of

taurine-high foods.)

6. *Tyramine*, which is present in cheeses, alcoholic drinks
   and other dietary items, increases blood pressure and promotes migraine headaches. (See Appendix for full listing
   of tyramine-high foods.)

7. *Several studies* done on celery have shown benefits to suf-
   ferers of certain diseases. A few years back, celery was
   found to be beneficial to those suffering with arthritis.

   Science News reported on research being done showing celery to be quite helpful to bring blood pressure down.
   There is a naturally produced chemical in celery which
   brings these beneficial results; it is 3-n-butyl phthalide. It
   widens blood vessels by relaxing the smooth muscle present
   in the walls of blood vessels. Three large stalks of celery
   ground in a blender yield about a glassful. Eight ounces of
   ground celery made fresh daily should supply enough
   phthalide to make a difference.[101] In one study done at the
   University of Chicago, those test subjects who took a single
   glassful per day of the ground celery for three months, had
   a 13% reduction in blood pressure.[102]

8. *Omega-3 fatty acids* may lower blood pressure.[103] Flaxseed contains generous quantities of omega-3 fatty acids.
   Two tablespoons of freshly ground flaxseed taken with a
   meal may have a beneficial effect on blood pressure. Grind
   the seed daily in a blender or in a seed mill and sprinkle on
   salads, fruit juice or cereal. It gives a pleasant, nutty flavor
   to foods. In some cultures, flaxseed is prized as a replace-
   ment for nuts. Lightly toast the seed to inactivate a factor
   which may interfere with vitamin B6 metabolism, and grind
   freshly to avoid the rapid development of a rancid change
   in omega-3 fatty acids.

9. *Garlic and onion* have been shown to benefit some people
   who have high blood pressure. Many people find garlic
   and onion to be pleasant foods and the treatment is enjoyable whether or not a benefit is gained from it. Use from

74   one to 10 cloves with a meal, raw, blended in juice or finely chopped in salads or soups. The garlic may be lightly steamed for two to four minutes, baked whole as a globe cluster in an oven at 350 degrees for 10-15 minutes or microwaved for one minute and 10-20 seconds. The garlic should not be overcooked, only long enough to make it begin to get limp, loosen its skin and get a bit translucent.

Alcohol

It is well known that alcohol is a poisonous or toxic substance and those using it get intoxicated. The poisonous effect is not only on the brain but on every cell alcohol touches. It damages the heart, the kidneys and the blood vessels. Many reports link the use of all alcoholic drinks to elevation of blood pressure.[104]

general conditions which elevate blood pressure

There are certain general body conditions known to have an elevating effect on blood pressure. These include advanced **pulmonary disease**, **snoring** accompanied by **sleep apnea** (periods of failure to breathe), longstanding high serum **uric acid**, high **blood sugar**, high **cholesterol** and other blood fats, including fats from recently eaten meals. But foods rich in fiber rather than added fats, and naturally high in magnesium and potassium will reduce blood pressure in most people.[105]

Uric acid is a waste product from foods high in purines. Purines are naturally occurring food substances usually found in foods also high in protein. When uric acid goes up in the blood it not only raises blood pressure but may cause gout and kidney trouble. Many foods high in protein are often high in purines as well. Animal products, meat, milk, eggs and cheese are the foods in American diets which are highest in proteins.

Blood fats are fats we obtain from the food we eat and those we manufacture in the body, principally in the liver. The fats we eat include free, or visible fats, and invisible fats.

76 Invisible fats are fats that are bound with proteins, carbohydrates, mineral and vitamin complexes in a natural association in unrefined foods. These other bound nutrients determine the rate at which the fats are used and the location where they will be deposited, either in arteries, hips or in the liver to be used in vital processes. But free fats have been separated from other nutrients bound to them by forcing them apart with food refining equipment. Once isolated, fats lose the modifying influences of these other nutrients, become less water soluble and are generally more hazardous to your health.

Invisible fats are found in peanuts, grains, olives, avocados, beans, nuts and seeds as well as many other foods. Free fats are found in margarine, butter, mayonnaise, fried foods, cooking fats, salad oils and nut butters such as peanut butter and tahini.

Apo - Lipoprotein

The outside shell possesses ports for attachment of the apo-lipoprotein. These lipoproteins are address labels for delivery to special sites, and differ for different forms of fats, free or invisible.

Fat goes to the duodenum (the beginning portion of the small intestine) for certain steps in digestion and for address labeling. The address labels mark the fat particles so that they know where to land as they float by various organs in the blood stream. The address label for free fats is made of apoprotein and is different from the label for invisible fats. When free fat goes to the duodenum the body handles it in a different way than if it were an invisible fat. Free fats are more difficult to process and transport, and the actual work of processing has an adverse effect on blood pressure.

Eating pork, even unsalted, can bring on high blood pressure.[106] The flesh of swine is high in purines, high in saturated fats, and naturally high in sodium, the harmful factor in salt.

Allergies of various kinds can raise blood pressure in some people. In the susceptible individual, both airborne and ingested allergens will cause an elevation of blood pressure. Since the 1930's a relationship has been recognized in some people, between certain foods and high blood pressure. It would be helpful to you to undertake an elimination and challenge diet to try and discover foods that may have an effect on your blood pressure. Simply leave a food out of your diet for three months and see if it makes a difference in your blood pressure; then try another food.

The most favorable diet for people with high blood pressure is a simple vegan diet--fruits, vegetables, whole grains and a few nuts and seeds. Breakfast should be principally fruit and whole grains and lunch should be mainly vegetables and whole grains. Either or both meals can have one or two tablespoons of nuts or seeds. Use fewer of these high calorie foods if you are overweight.

Fruit, either raw or preserved in some way other than with salt, vinegar or sugar, has been found to help people with high blood pressure or increased uric acid. [107, 108] Weight control helps the blood pressure. [109, 110]

Since overweight, particularly of the abdomen or trunk, is now known to be related not only to hypertension but also to heart disease, cancer and diabetes, it is not surprising to find that the same factors which work to alleviate diabetes, also help decrease high blood pressure. These are diet, exercise, weight control and support groups to help people stay with the program.

Numerous studies show that, in general, the more overweight the person, the more likely to develop hypertension.

78   Even if the obese person does not have high blood pressure, he is much more likely to develop it, along with insulin resistance, within the ensuing 10 years.

Studies are also showing that weight loss, even no more than 10–15 pounds, if sustained, will have a significantly beneficial effect on hypertension.

Contemporary weight charts are generally not adequate to use when judging your own weight, because they are based on American averages. These averages do not take the level of health into consideration; they are figures of what has been found to be an average weight for thousands of people, both sick and well. Considering that most people are eating food that will raise their blood pressures, are obviously carrying excess rolls of fat and are not exercising, these figures are not ones you want to base your weight on.

To emphasize that these averages are not necessarily ones to follow, studies have proven that for people in the same age group, those of average weight die earlier than those who are a few pounds lighter. If a man is 10% above his desirable weight, his mortality rate is 11% higher. A woman who is 10% above her ideal weight will have a 6% higher mortality rate. [120]

So what is the ideal weight? For people in perfect health it may be adequate to figure the weight by allowing 100 pounds for the first five feet. Then add five pounds per inch above five feet for women, and six to seven pounds per inch for men, depending on how muscular they are. But for people with serious health problems, it may be desirable to figure the weight by the following formula: Multiply your height in inches by 3.5 for women and by 4.0 for men. Subtract 108 from the result for women and 128 for men. The end figure will often be 10-20 per cent lower than the first formula will give. Many people will fare much better at a lighter weight.

Set Points for Weight Control

Set points are established limits for body structures, processes and chemical levels. A set point is a level the weight control devices of the body see as the "normal," and will adjust metabolism, and the appetite to maintain that level, even if it is far above the ideal. We have many hundreds of set points in the body, from the length hair will grow before it falls out to how high blood proteins are. Once a set point has been broken, there may be rapid changes in others, such as cholesterol, blood sugar, weight and blood pressure. There are controlling factors which cause the set point to go up or down. We will discuss those factors which make the set point for weight slide continually upward.

Factors That Affect Set Points for Weight

1. The more free fat one eats, the higher the set point for weight. Free fats are fats detached from carbohydrates, proteins, minerals or vitamins (see #1 in the "Program Guidelines" list in Chapter Eleven for a discussion of free fats; see the Index for other listings). Saturated fat, which is generally animal fat, will raise the set point more than unsaturated fat from plant sources.
2. Eating between meals raises the set point. This factor will be intensified if snacks contain free fats. Unfortunately, snacks are more likely to contain free fats. Furthermore, studies show that the calories you eat between meals are less likely to keep your appetite under control than if you eat the same number of calories at your meal.[121]
3. Regular, moderate exercise will lower the set points.
4. A sedentary lifestyle increases set points for weight, blood pressure and blood cholesterol.
5. Irregular meal times raises set points.
6. Eating sweets raises the set points. The digestion of sweets has a specific metabolic effect which, although it is similar to that of eating free fats, it is not as influential in

raising the set points as are free fats.

7. Loss of sleep increases the set point for weight although it may allow temporary weight loss.

8. Green, leafy vegetables, salads, fruits and whole grains reduce the set points.

9. Late and heavy suppers raise the set point.

10. Protein of animal origin raises the set points by the growth promotion factor. (See #2 in the "Program Guidelines" list in Chapter Eleven for further discussion of the growth factor.)

11. People who use coffee, tea, colas or chocolate have been shown to have a higher body mass index (overweight).

12. Eating food or nourishing drinks after about 3:00 p.m. will raise the set points. For reasons not well understood, eating after 3:00 p.m. causes the body to believe it should build a bigger warehouse to store additional nutrients. Up goes the set point for weight!

13. Short-term fasting (a day or two a week) tends to lower the set point.

HYPERTENSION DIET

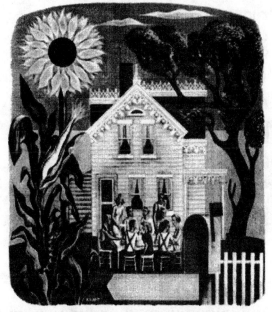

Mini Cookbook

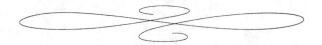

CONTENTS

Cracker Recipes

ROLLED OAT CRACKERS

1¼ c. quick oats
⅓ c. unsweetened coconut
1 T. whole grain flour
¼ t. salt (*omit while blood pressure high*)
⅓ c. cold water

Blend first four ingredients until fine. Pour into mixing bowl and add water. Mix well. Roll onto an oiled cookie sheet very thin, ⅛" and score. Bake at 250 to 325 for 15-20 minutes. Watch carefully and remove the thinnest crackers as soon as browned.

CORN FRITOS

1½ c. cornmeal
3 c. hot boiling water
1 t. salt (omit)
2 T. oil (omit)

Put ingredients into a mixing bowl and pour boiling water in, mixing well. Pour onto two 10 x 15" oiled cookie sheets. Distribute evenly by tilting sheets from side to side. Bake at 350 for 20 minutes.

Remove from oven and score into frito strips. Bake again at 250–300 watching carefully and removing the thinnest fritos around the edges as soon as done.

SUNNY OAT CRACKERS

3 c. oat flour (*see instructions below*)
1 ¼ c. water
1 ½ t. salt (*omit*)
¾ c. sunflower seeds

Put about 2½ cups of rolled or quick oats in a blender and grind until a uniform flour. It may take more oats to make three cups. Do not pack the flour. Set aside in a mixing bowl. No need to rinse blender, put the seeds, salt (omit), and a portion of the water in the blender until smooth. Mix all ingredients in the bowl and knead well for smoothness and flakiness (five minutes in a mixer is perfect, but can be done by hand). Put a ¾" ball of dough between two layers of kitchen plastic, or use a dough press as for tortillas, and roll out very thin. Bake for 10 minutes at 350 or until crisp. Watch carefully to prevent burning.

Dairy Product Substitutes
Cheeses

CASHEW CHEESE SAUCE
For broccoli, potatoes, or grilled cheese sandwiches

¾ c. rinsed cashews
2 T. sesame seeds
2 t. onion powder
⅛ - ¾ t. garlic powder
1 c. water
1¼ t. salt (*omit*)
2 T. lemon juice
½ c. pimentos
⅛ t. dill weed (opt.)
¼ c. quick oats

Blend ingredients till smooth. Cook till thickened.
Use the quick oats only if to be used for sandwiches.

SLICING CHEESE
(*get plant gel and millet at health food store*)

Soak the following in blender two to three minutes:
½ c. cold water
3 T. Emes gel

Add and blend until smooth the following:
¼ c. cashews
¼ c. chopped onion
1 c. hot cooked millet
2 T. lemon juice
1 garlic clove
⅓ c. pimento
1½ t. salt (*omit*)

Pour into a pan to mold. Refrigerate 4 hours. Slice.

GARBANZO CHEESE

Soak 1 cup dry garbanzos for 24 hours. Sprout 48 hours. Rinse every 12 hours. Then blend smooth:

½ c. nuts or sunflower seed
¼ c. lemon juice
2 c. sprouted garbanzos
½ c. pimentos
1 c. water
1½ t. onion powder
1½ t. salt (*omit*)
⅛-½ t. garlic powder

Pour into oiled loaf pan. Bake 1½ hours at 350. Cool. Remove from pan. Slice.

JACK CHEESE

Soak for 3-4 minutes the following:
1 c. cold water
6–7 T. Emes gelatin
Pour in 1½ c. boiling water, blend and cool slightly:

Add and blend the following:

2 c. cashews
½ c. yeast flakes
1 T. salt (*omit*)
2 t. onion powder
½ c. lemon juice
½ to 1 t. garlic powder
3 T. finely grated carrot or cooked carrot for color.

Pour into a loaf pan to mold it. Cool slightly. Cover

and refrigerate overnight or 4 hours till firm.

AMERICAN CHEESE

Use the above recipe for Jack Cheese, but use ¼ cup less of boiling water, and half the amount of yeast flakes, lemon juice and garlic powder. Cover before refrigerating.

CREAM CHEESE

Soak several minutes:
2 T. Emes unflavored gel
⅓ c. water
Add and blend: ½ c. boiling water
Add and blend: 1 c. raw cashews
Add and blend: 2-3 c. firm tofu (*may need to blend half at a time as it gets quite thick*)
2 t. salt (*omit*)
Refrigerate in a loaf pan until firm.

SESAME CREAM CHEESE

¼ c. sesame seed
½ t. onion powder
2 T. cornstarch
¼ t. garlic powder
1 c. water
2 T. lemon juice
½ t. salt (*omit*)
Seasonings*

Blend ingredients except seasonings* (chives and parsley, fresh and chopped fine are suggestions). Heat until thickened. Cool mixture. Add chives and parsley or other herbs to your taste. Chill and serve.

COTTAGE CHEESE

1 lb. firm tofu
¼ t. garlic powder
½ t. lemon juice
¼ t. onion powder
1 t. salt (*omit*)
½ c. cashews

Rinse and crumb ¾ of the tofu. Blend the remaining tofu with rest of the ingredients. Add enough water to make it creamy and stir into the crumbled tofu. Chill and use in any way you need.

GOLDEN SAUCE

¾ c. water
½ t. salt (*omit*)
½ c. potatoes
1 to 3 T. lemon juice
¼ c. carrots (*for color*)*
1 to 2 T. nuts or seeds
1 to 2 T. food yeast

Liquefy ingredients in blender until smooth. Cook only if potatoes and carrots are raw. Heat to serving temperature and serve over rice, grits, macaroni, vegetables, broccoli, greens, and vegetarian roasts. *Tomatoes or pimentos may be used instead of carrots. Cooked rice, millet or spaghetti may be substituted for potatoes.

MELTY CHEESE

2 c. water
1¾ t. salt (*omit*)
⅔ c. cashews
1½ t. onion powder
½ c. food yeast
½ t. garlic powder
¼ c. cooked carrots
1 t. butter flavor (*opt*)
3 T. pimentos
¼ t. dill weed
1 T. tomato sauce (*opt*)
2 T. arrowroot powder
1 T. fresh lemon juice
¼ c. cornstarch

Blend all ingredients at medium speed for two minutes. Let rest three minutes. Blend again at high speed for two minutes. Stir, while cooking on low heat until thickened. Simmer gently about two more minutes. Serve hot over baked potatoes or pasta, immediately after cooking. Left over cheese may be chilled and used as a spread for toast, crackers, or sandwiches. Very good with celery sticks or in chili beans.

Butters

NUT OR SEED BUTTER

Blend until smooth:
1 c. nuts or seeds, any kind
½ c. water
¼ t. salt (*omit*)

If you like commercial nut butters like peanut butter, then you will want to roast the nuts or seeds at 275 until light brown. Butters can be made from raw nuts or seeds, also. Grind in a blender or seed mill to a fine powder if you want the very smoothest butter. Add ¼ to ½ cup of water as needed to turn blender blades. Use a rubber spatula to keep the nuts off the sides and against the blender blades. If the butter becomes too liquid while you are blending it, simply add more nuts as needed to adjust the consistency. Experience will tell you how much water is needed for each type of nut or seed.

CORN BUTTER
(or Millet or Rice Butter)

Blend until very smooth:
½ c. coconut
½ t. salt (*omit*)
½ c. hot water
½ t. lemon extract

Add and blend until very smooth about one cup or more of hot, well-cooked cornmeal, whole kernel corn or grits. May use well cooked millet or rice instead of corn.

DRIED FRUIT BUTTER

Apple butter: Put applesauce in a large flat pan in the oven to concentrate at 250 for several hours. When evaporation has left a thick paste, put into a storage container. Keeps several weeks in refrigerator. Vanilla or coriander also may be added.

Pear butter: Use canned pears. Liquefy in blender. Process as for apple butter. Any canned fruit or berry may be treated in this manner for delicious, nutritious spreads of low calorie content.

Apricot butter: To two-thirds cup of stewed, dried apricots, add enough pineapple juice or orange juice (about equal quantity as the apricots) in a blender to make a thick butter. Add lemon juice if not tart enough, or juice concentrate if not sweet enough. Any dried fruit may be used for butter.

Cream

SESAME-COCONUT CREAM

2 c. boiling water
½ c. grated fresh coconut (*may use dry, unsweet-
     ened shredded coconut*)
1 t. honey (*omit*)
½ c. sesame seed
¼ t. salt (*omit*)

Liquefy and serve. May be strained if a smoother
texture is desired. Dilute if necessary.

NUT CREAM

To one cup of water in the blender, add about half
quantity of nuts or seeds, more if the nuts or seeds have
been roasted, less if the nuts are fresh from the trees as
theey blend smoother. Generally nuts and seeds are not
roasted for creams, but a very pleasant cream can be
made from lighted toasted nuts. Roast the nuts or seeds
by spreading on a large, flat pan in the oven at 250 for
several hours. Test occasionally, as oven temperatures
vary greatly. Salt is used in the commercial creams, but
may be omitted in home prepared creams.

SOUR CREAM

Add two to six tablespoons of lemon juice to any
nut or seed butter, or tofu mayonnaise. Optional seasonings: Onion powder, garlic powder, dill weed,
chopped chives or parsley, dried onion or garlic flakes.

Mayonnaise

TOFU MAYONNAISE

Blend until creamy smooth:
1 c. tofu
½ c. water
2 T. lemon juice
4 T. sesame seed
2 t. onion powder
1 t. honey (omit)
½ t. garlic powder
½ t. salt (omit)

HUMMUS
(a favorite!)

2 c. cooked garbanzos
½-¾ c. sesame seed
3-7 T. lemon juice
1 clove garlic
1 T. chopped parsley (opt.)
Salt (omit)
⅓ c. bean juice, or more
  onion and garlic powder to taste

Blend together until smooth. Serve in sandwiches, on zwieback, baked potatoes, rice, spaghetti, salad, or use as dip for vegetables. Very versatile spread.

SUNFLOWER MAYONNAISE

Bring to a boil:
1 c. water
½ c. sunflower seed

Blend well with:
½ c. well cooked millet*
1 t. garlic powder
¼ t. dill weed
1 t. onion powder
¼ c. lemon juice
¼ c. cashews (*opt.*)
½ t. salt (*omit*)

*Note: Millet may be substituted by an equal quantity of well cooked rice or two to three baked potatoes.

Ice Cream

BANANA ICE CREAM

Select very ripe bananas, peel, freeze. Break or cut bananas into six to twelve pieces. Put in blender with barely enough pineapple juice, (orange or apple juice may be used) to blend--about ¼ to ½ cup, more or less. Should be soft- serve consistency. Serve over waffles, cereal, hard toast, fresh fruit or berries, or even hot oatmeal.

FRUTARI

2 c. crushed pineapple, drained
12 oz can frozen apple juice concentrate
2 or 3 dates (*opt.*)
3 T. Emes unflavored gel
1 c. pineapple juice

Put the last two ingredients in a sauce pan and bring to a boil to dissolve. Set off stove to cool. Blend the crushed pineapple and dates until smooth. Mix everything together. Freeze. Blenderize or put through a Champion juicer. More gelatin can be added to make it creamier if desired.

CAROB ICE CREAM (CHOCOLATE-LIKE)

5 dates
½-¾ c. water
¼ t. salt (*omit*)
½ c. cashews
2 T. carob powder
1½ t. vanilla
4-6 frozen bananas

Blend all ingredients except the bananas until it is very smooth. Use the smallest amount of water to keep the blender blades turning. Cut bananas into eight to twelve pieces each and add a few at a time until you have made the mixture about the consistency of soft-serve ice cream.

Milks

NUT MILK--BASIC RECIPE FOR ANY NUT OR SEED

Blend until very smooth:
1 c. nuts
1 c. water
salt (*omit*), honey (*omit*), and vanilla if desired

Then add:
2 to 3 c. water to adjust consistency as desired

TOFU MILK

Blend until creamy:
1 c. tofu
½ c. water

Add to blender
2 t. vanilla (*opt*)
½ t. salt (*omit*)
1 T. honey (*omit*)
1 c. water

Continue adding water to desired consistency, usually about 2¾ to 4 more cups.

LEMON COCONUT MILK

Blend very smooth, adding liquid little by little
½ c. hot cooked cereal, rice, millet, barley, etc.
½ c. coconut, ground fine in blender or seed mill
½ t. lemon extract
1½ c. hot water
1½ c. hot pineapple juice
Good over cereal.

CAROB MILK SHAKE

4 c. nut milk
1 or 2 ripe bananas
3 T. carob powder
½ t. salt (*omit*)
1 T. unsweetened shredded coconut

Blend thoroughly. Chill or heat to serve. To use this milkshake with a vegetable meal, substitute bananas with three-quarter cup of baked sweet potato or butternut or other sweet winter squash.

Dips and Spreads

For Sandwiches, Potatoes, Toast, Rolls, Bread Sticks, Crackers, or Finger Foods and Relish Items

AVOCADO DIP OR SPREAD

2 c. mashed ripe avocado
½ t. garlic powder
1½ T. lemon juice
1½ t. onion powder
¾ t. salt (*omit*)

Mix together, and may serve as is. You may want to add one-half cup of any mayonnaise you have made, and/or one cup finely minced tomatoes.

HERB DIP

Add to either your own mayonnaise or sour cream about one tablespoon of basil or dill. Use any cheese for which we have given recipes above, any butter, or hummus as a spread or dip.

OLIVE SPREAD OR DIP

1 lb firm tofu, cubed
½ c. chopped olives
3 T. food yeast
½ c. tofu mayonnaise
1½ T. lemon juice, fresh
Salt (*omit*)
1½ t. onion powder
⅛ t. garlic powder
Pinch dill weed

Rinse and drain tofu well. Cube rather finely. Put in a mixing bowl with remaining ingredients, except mayonnaise, and mix well. Mix in the mayonnaise, chill and use with lettuce or onion slices to make sandwiches, or serve with dinner rolls.

Cakes

WAFFLE CAKE

4 waffles with 4 squares each
1 c. sunflower seeds or nuts, finely chopped
1 recipe carob sauce (page 102)
Banana ice cream* from eight bananas or more
Sliced bananas for top (*optional*), and unsweet
    ened shredded coconut for garnish (*optional*).

Ahead of time, freeze waffles flat on a large cookie
sheet. Have all ingredients chilled. Work fast to prevent much melting. Lay one waffle on a large flat plat-
ter with plenty of room on all sides to catch runoff ice
cream. Spoon one or two tablespoons of carob sauce
on each square of the waffle. Spread with a knife.
Spread about ½ to ¾" of banana ice cream on sauce
to make the layer. Sprinkle with about one- quarter cup
of chopped nuts. Place second waffle on the ice cream
and repeat the layers in any order you prefer. After all
four layers have been made, "ice" the cake with the
remainder of the ice cream or carob sauce. Slice bananas on top to garnish. Sprinkle with the coconut.
Put the cake in the freezer for it to set—about one hour.
Remove, slice with a sharp knife, using care not to dis-
turb the layers. *Instead of banana ice cream and carob
sauce, a dried fruit butter, chopped nuts, and a cream
cheese may be used to make the layers with the waffles.
Do not put in freezer, but set in refrigerator for it to set
before slicing.

UNCOOKED FRUIT CAKE

1 c. raisins, ground
1 c. dates, chopped
2 c. diced mixed dried fruit
3 T. cornstarch
1 c. fruit juice concentrate
¾ c. fruit juice
1 c. sunflower seed or nuts
1 c. whole wheat bread crumbs

Put the juice concentrate, the fruit juice and the cornstarch together in a saucepan and heat until starch is clear. Pour it into a mixing bowl with the bread crumbs and wet them thoroughly. Add all other ingredients and toss together. Pack into a loaf pan or casserole dish. Do not cut for 1-2 days. Cut carefully to prevent breaking it up.

Sauces

FRESH FRUIT SAUCE

Put two peeled, quartered and cored apples and two peeled and deseeded oranges in the blender together, putting the orange in first. Blend the orange and add the apple quarters or eighths and blend to sauce consistency. Fresh blueberries, blackberries, raspberries or strawberries may be blended for a delicious berry sauce.

BLUEBERRY SAUCE OR TOPPING

12 oz frozen unsweetened grape juice
12 oz water
¼ c. plus 1 T. tapioca or cornstarch
1 box frozen blueberries, or 1-3 c. fresh berries

Mix tapioca and liquids and let set for 4 minutes. Heat and simmer about three to five minutes until tapioca is dissolved, stirring frequently. Remove from heat and cool a few minutes. Stir in blueberries.

CAROB TOPPING

1 c. nut milk
3 T. cornstarch
8-15 dates
1 t. vanilla
¼ c. carob powder
½ t. salt (*omit*)

Stir or blend all ingredients until smooth. Bring to a boil, stirring until thick, about ten minutes. Pour into serving dish, cover and chill. Sprinkle shredded unsweetened coconut for garnish over top.

CAROB SAUCE

1 c. water
2-4 T. starch
2 t. vanilla
2 T. carob powder
4-10 dates
3 T. pecans
⅛ t. salt (*omit*)

Mix ingredients in blender. Cook until starch is thickened. Adjust the consistency by adding more or less starch. Serve over waffles, use in the waffle cake, use as a topping for banana ice cream or spread on crackers or rolls.

Pickles

PICKLES WITHOUT VINEGAR

8 c. water
2 c. lemon juice
¼ c. pickling salt (*omit*)
Fresh cucumbers

Set to boil. Meanwhile put one teaspoon of dill seed in all clean quart jars you plan to fill with pickles. Pack tightly with clean cucumbers (whole, sliced or spears). Add one to two tablespoons of dried onion chips or freshly chopped onions, two teaspoons of dehydrated garlic, as well as several whole cloves of garlic if you like lots of garlic. Put two sprigs of dill weed in the sides of jars if you like the fronded appearance, and a second teaspoon of dill seed on the tops of the cucumbers. When the solution is boiling, fill the jars to the neck with the boiling lemon water. Adjust quantities of seasonings for pints and half-gallons.
Process in a water bath canner:

Half-gallons	-	10 minutes
Quarts	-	8 minutes
Pints	-	5 minutes

section
three

ways to treat hypertension

104

Case History

The successful use of a very simple program to control blood pressure is illustrated by the following case. This case also shows how people are often resistant at first, or even afraid of the unknown in lifestyle change.

MB, the mother of a Seventh-day Adventist minister was herself a Southern Baptist and not interested in her son's careful health habits, but very sick with her blood pressure and the medications she took to try to bring it down. She resisted strongly her son's efforts to get her to see a physician in his church. Finally she agreed to see me as I was only visiting for a few weeks in the town and would not pose a long term threat to her aversion to lifestyle change. Yet she was resentful for the time spent to see me, and adamant to me that she would "not go to the hospital." She was deeply depressed, felt she was at the end of life at age 55, and no force could change that. She did not want to spend one penny more than necessary to buy her medicines, so she could leave her estate intact for her children and many grandchildren. She expected to die anytime, and life had become a burden. She weighed over 200 pounds and could not budge her weight from there.

As she entered the room where I was set up to do her physical she was complaining to her daughter-in-law, a registered nurse, how doctors were so expensive. Her daughter-in-law explained that I was a dear friend and expected no fee from her. I began her physical examination with other observations than her blood pressure, and was about half finished before I applied the blood pressure cuff. I was shocked with the reading.

I said, "Mary, you must go immediately to Uchee Pines for treatment of your blood pressure."

"I told you I am not going to the hospital," she exploded. Her daughter-in-law explained to her that Uchee Pines is not a hospital. But she was determined.

106

"How high is it, anyway?" she demanded.
I said, "240/140."

"Why, that's no higher than it has been for the last year!"

She removed from a handbag her large medical record which supported what she had said--not a single reading during the past year below 240/140. She assured me she never missed a dose of her medicines, three of the most powerful known for blood pressure.

I explained to her my reluctance to undertake her case as an outpatient, that we needed her to be under constant supervision and a consistently reliable program directed by someone who would be strict with everything.

Her daughter-in-law said very cryptically, "Mother **will** follow everything you say!"

I could hear enough determination in that voice that I agreed to help her under one condition: she must follow my program to the letter. She agreed. I wrote out three pages of instructions: start with a three day total food fast, 12 glasses of water each day, four of which could be hawthorne berry tea. The next three days would be an apple fast, using only apples for food for three meals, followed by a dairy-, eggs-, salt-, and fat-free vegetarian diet. Her blood pressure and weight must be monitored daily. She should soak in a warm tub 30 minutes twice a day. She must take a stroll in the cool of the day, both morning and evening. Her daughter-in-law must call me daily with a report. She should have a foot massage or backrub every evening before bedtime. I cautioned her to faithfully take her blood pressure medicines.

Frankly, I did not believe the daily reports I got from her daughter-in-law which indicated a falling blood pressure from the first day. But when she returned in a week she had lost 12 pounds and had a blood pressure of 198/102! She was remarkably different in attitude. Now she was of quiet demeanor, looked cheerful and cooperative; her face was not bloated; she had no agitated depression as formerly, and several times she said incredulously, "Nobody ever told me how to get my blood pressure down." The next week she decided on her own to stop taking her blood pressure medicines.

When she returned to see me with a further drop in blood pressure, I said, "We can start tapering off your medicines now."

"Oh, I dropped those last week!", she said triumphantly. I must have looked shocked. Then I did some serious instruction.

"You must never just drop blood pressure medicine. It is dangerous not to taper it off, as the blood pressure can jump very high in a rebound."

She said, "They weren't doing any good anyway, and just made me depressed and forgetful." I could not deny that!

Mary lost 50 pounds and her blood pressure came down to 112/78, and has stayed down for the past eleven years every time I have inquired about her. She still maintains her lifestyle changes.

108

forty days to reverse hypertension

Healing, Restoring, Regaining Health – Without Using Drugs

We can regard inherited degenerative disease to be a form of accelerated aging. This includes overweight, diabetes, hardening of the arteries, hypertension, and laboratory evidence of aging such as high blood levels of cholesterol, sugar, uric acid, urea nitrogen, and iron. You can trim this list down to size. In 40 days you can establish a new lifestyle that does not promote those diseases that destroy the quality of life of most retirees.

The 40 Day Health Recovery Program

Sixty million Americans have some degree of hypertension; probably 90 percent or more of these could be cured simply by following the Health Recovery Program. Follow the program for a full year before making any deviations. Then a small change occasionally of certain items, such as salt or honey may be well tolerated. Faithfully continue the exercise, diet, regularity and other good health measures as long as you live. Signs of premature aging indicate an urgent need for the program.

110

Signs and Symptoms of Premature Aging
These signs and symptoms have been shown to be associated with an accelerated rate of aging. While not applicable to all people, they can give some clues to those whose situation is not the most ideal.

Findings in Your History and Physical
Acne
Allergies
Appendectomy
Arthritis
Birth weight over 8 pounds
Cataracts before 60
Diabetes
Dizziness, persistent
Headaches
Heart rate over 80
Low resistance to disease with frequent colds,
  sore throats, boils, skin or nail problems
More than 5 fillings by age 20
More than 5 teeth missing by age 30
Overweight
Peptic Ulcer
Rapid growth in early childhood
Sleep loss, chronic
Slow healing
Tonsillectomy

Laboratory Reports Out of Ideal Range:
  Glucose not 70-85
  BUN above 15
  Thyroid not 4-12
  Sodium above 140
  Cholesterol above 100 + age
  WBC above 6,000

Triglycerides above 100
Hemoglobin levels out of ideal ranges:
Female: 10.5- 12.5
Male: 12.0- 14.75
Uric acid above 5
Serum iron above 80

As you look at this list, notice that these are all signs of eating too much of something (or everything!). Therefore it is logical we should begin recovery by—

Fasting

Fasting is a beneficial way to gain appetite control, help accustom yourself to the tastes of more healthful foods, restore function of insulin receptors as discussed in Chapter Three, and help you lose any extra weight. Prolonged fasting for more than three days every week can be damaging, while short term fasting of one or two meals, or even one or two days, can be useful.

Fasting can be done easily by omitting supper on day one and all meals on day two. On day three, the fast can be broken by eating one-quarter the size of the usual breakfast, one-half the usual lunch, and no supper. On day four, three-quarters of the usual breakfast can be eaten. Lunch on day four will be the first full meal after the fast. Spend as many hours breaking the fast as were spent in the fast.

Fasting is not only a good way to gain control of the appetite, it helps directly to control blood pressure, diabetes and blood fats.

FOODS ALLOWED DURING 40 DAYS

Main Dishes

A vegetarian diet is best. However, if meat and eggs are eaten, they should be overcooked to try and kill germs and cancer viruses, and then meat should be blotted to remove

112   excess fat. Limit their use in accordance with the recommendations of the American Heart Association to two to five times a week, except for objectionable meats such as seafood, pork, ham, bacon, sausage, hot dogs, hamburger, canned meat spreads, pressed meats, and canned composite meats such as Spam, which should all be permanently eliminated. There are acceptable commercial meat substitutes, although meat substitutes may be too high in protein and free fats to be the most healthful.

Dairy milk products are not recommended for hypertensives. Milk sensitivity is the commonest form of food sensitivity in the United States. Many signs, such as elevated blood pressure, that have obscure or unknown causes could have their origin in the use of milk. It is always worth a three month trial off milk products. If you find you are sensitive to milk, eliminating milk permanently will have lasting benefits.

Quick and easy blender-made nut milks, also soy milk made from soybeans (commercial soy milks are usually heavily sweetened and filled with free fats), cheeses made from nuts, flours or vegetables, and sour and sweet creams made from special recipes are all recommended as milk substitutes. These milks may be used in cooking and with meals. You may use green or black olives (not stuffed) and avocado prepared attractively and tastily for butter and cheese substitutes. See recipes in Chapter Fourteen.

Nuts and Seeds

If shelled nuts are purchased, they need to be cooked or sterilized if eaten raw. To sterilize: wash the shelled raw nuts in cool water and heat them in the oven at 225 degrees until dry, stirring occasionally.

Cheese

There are cheeses, butters and sauces made from nuts, potatoes, carrots, tomatoes, onions, other vegetables and seasonings to make tasty creams, spreads and dips for vegetables, pastas and breads. Simple and inexpensive dishes are made from appropriate recipes. See sources for *Eat For Strength, Oil–Free* cookbook, and recipes in Chapter Fourteen.

Breads

Use only whole grain breads. Two of three grains may be mixed for a single bread. Bread should be thoroughly cooked and well chewed.

Cereals

Use only whole grain cereals. Commercial cream of wheat is not a whole grain. If you like cream of wheat, substitute bulgar wheat or farina, or use the recipe in *Eat For Strength* cookbook (available from New Lifestyle Books) for cream of wheat using whole kernel wheat. You may also make cream of rice, cream of corn or cream of any whole grain. Some other easily prepared whole grain cereals are oatmeal, steel- cut oats, granola (without oil or honey), wheat cereals, buckwheat, barley, millet, grits or whole wheat macaroni. Soy spaghetti is also acceptable.

Vegetables

Vegetables may be used in liberal quantities. When used in the menu as a vegetable rather than as a main dish, the very starchy vegetables such as Irish potatoes, corn, spaghetti, macaroni, sweet potatoes, or dried beans should be restricted to about 100 calorie portions, If corn, rice, spaghetti, macaroni, potatoes, or dried beans and peas are used as a main dish, a single serving should contain 250 to 300 calories. Very active people, young men and pregnant or lactating mothers may need seconds.

Coffee and Tea Substitutes

Coffee, tea, colas and chocolate have all been found to cause an elevation of blood pressure. All beverage herb teas are acceptable substitutes: lemon grass, lemon mint, etc. Postum, Cafix, Pero and other commercial coffee and tea substitutes are also acceptable, but some of these types of beverages have molasses or sugar beet residues in them. Check

114 labels carefully and avoid these if you have tendencies toward diabetes as well.

Artificial Sweeteners

It is best to learn to eat foods in their natural, unsweetened state as much as possible. One should cultivate the habit of not using sweeteners.

Satisfy your sweet tooth with an abundance of fruit, which even diabetics can use. Check out the unusual ones at markets catering to foreign customers. All fresh fruits, canned in water pack or natural juices may be used.

Remember that fruit juices should be made fresh for the best nourishment. Refined juices, such as canned and bottled ones, are not fresh and there is no fiber to help them to digest.

FOODS TO AVOID

Sugars, Condiments and Salt

Until the blood pressure and the laboratory test results are in the ideal range, all white, brown or raw sugar, fructose, honey, syrups, jams, jellies, preserves, Jell-O, etc., salt, soy sauce, commercial sauces and condiments, chips and nuts unless fat and salt–free, should be eliminated from the diet. Read all labels. Many of these foods have generous supplies of heavy or unwieldy nutrients which can be thought of as having irritating qualities for the heart and arteries. The chronic injury is what causes the acceleration of aging for susceptible persons.

Bear in mind that many medicines have quite a lot of salt, sugar or other nutrients which are difficult for the body to handle. As an example, Zantac–the most popular pharmaceutical of our day–in tablet form has no salt, but in the effervescent tablet there are 370 milligrams.

Avoid spices, black and hot pepper, commercial mayonnaise and catsup, vinegar and smoked or salt–cured foods. Home–canned pickles are essentially canned cucumbers and may be prepared healthfully from a good recipe using lemon juice and salt. See *Eat For Strength* cookbook and pickle recipe in Chapter Fourteen.

Breads, Pastries and Pastas

All pies, cakes, sweetened desserts, Jell-O, which is only sweetened, colored, flavored water with a small amount of gelatin (a refined protein), need to be avoided. Learn to make your own pies and cakes healthfully from a good cookbook like Eat For Strength.

Crackers, cakes and cookies become unhealthful when made with baking soda or powder, eggs, milk, shortening, and some flavorings, colorings and conditioners. Avoid all granolas made with sugar, honey or oil, and all boxed cereals, unless free of salt and sugar. Crackers, cakes and cookies can be homemade healthfully. Recipes can be found in *Eat for Strength* cookbook. The whole grain pastas require a little longer cooking, but with a bit of practice, you will be able to handle these products just as well as the white flours. See cracker recipes in Chapter Fourteen.

Sweet Fruits

All dried fruits (raisins, dates, figs, etc.) should be eaten in moderation, as they are more concentrated than fresh fruit. It is easy to overeat dried fruit and overload the body with too much food. Overeating promotes accelerated aging.

Drinks

Avoid coffee (even Sanka and Decaff), tea, cola and other soft drinks and chocolate. All members of this group cause problems of one kind or another. Soft drinks include Kool-Aid, bottled drinks, etc. Fruit juices may be used as part of the fluid in recipes and for meals, but in large quantities these juices interfere with digestion, and cause insulin levels to rise higher than with fresh fruits..

Medicines Containing Caffeine

Some medicines also contain caffeine. These include Anacin, A.P.C., B.C., Caffergot, Cope, Coricidin, Dolor,

Empirin Compound, Excedrin, Fiorinal, 4-Way Cold Tablets, Stanback, Trigesic, Vanquish and many others.

Summary of Some General Principles

Eat a substantial breakfast and lunch. Supper, if eaten, should be only about 100 to 300 calories of whole grains or fruit. We have found that the two meal plan (breakfast and lunch, no supper) allows the body the greatest opportunity for recovery from the heavy work of digestion. There should be at least five hours between meals.

Do not vary mealtime from day to day if possible. Chew well. Blood sugar levels in rapid eaters fluctuate more widely than in those who eat slowly, and chew their food well.

Fluctuating blood sugar levels promote hypertension as well as diabetes. Do not allow a disease to make you neurotic or self- centered, to brood over supposed ills and to dwell on physical or emotional symptoms. Handle disease with a calm attitude, and trust that God will give you wisdom to supply all your needs.

Never eat between meals or take a bedtime snack. These practices are harmful to the body and accelerate aging.

Legumes (beans, peas, peanuts, etc.) potatoes, other root vegetables, okra, and the whole grains such as brown rice and pastas should be used as **main dishes** during the 40 days of the reverse hypertension program. These simple and inexpensive foods are excellent sources of nutrients and have the advantage of not raising blood pressure, blood cholesterol, sugar levels or endangering the health from animal diseases that are carried in animal products. They also tend to have about one-third less calories than lean meats.

Drink enough water between meals to keep the urine almost colorless. For most people, this will be six to eight glasses a day. Ideally you should drink water no closer than about fifteen minutes before meals, and wait about thirty minutes or more after meals to resume drinking. Generally the less fluid taken with meals the better. Much weakness and

fatigue are due to compensatory water shifts and the dehydrated person is actually "wilted" even if no thirst is experienced.

Exercise is your best friend. Twenty minutes per day
is minimal; one hour daily is better, but on certain days you
may need three to five hours of physical activity. Do not get
sunburned and do not make your muscles sore with too much
exercise. These excesses are not healthful. Gradually build
to a good exercise level without developing sore muscles.
Exercise helps keep your appetite under control, neutralizes
stress, reduces blood pressure, lowers blood cholesterol, promotes digestion and normalizes blood sugar. Make it your
companion. Breathe deeply while exercising and meditate
on nature as you work out.

Elimination And Challenge Diet

The elimination and challenge diet should be used for
another 40 days if hypertension has not diminished after following the Health Recovery Program for 40 days. This per-
sistence of high blood pressure may indicate food allergies or
sensitivities, such as to gluten.

The best way to find out if you are allergic to foods is
simply omit certain foods you will be testing for a period of
time, usually three to six weeks. During this time certain
symptoms indicating a sensitivity to a food should disappear.
That tells you one or more of the foods you have eliminated
is the culprit. To find the foods involved in your problem,
begin adding back, one at a time every five to seven days, the
foods on the list. When a food causes your blood pressure to
go up, banish that food for a year. Then test it carefully again
to see if you can now tolerate it without raising your blood
pressure. Use the lists on the following pages for the test.

Check Yourself for Allergies to Foods on the next pages ☞

118

Foods to Avoid
Apples
Artificial food colors
Bananas
Beef
Beer, alcohol
Cane sugar
Chocolate
Cinnamon, ginger, nutmeg, hot pepper
Citrus fruits and juices
Coffee
Colas
Corn–cornstarch, corn products
Dairy products (cause over 60% of allergies)
Eggs
Fish
Garlic
Legumes, peanuts, soybean products
Lettuce
Nightshades–eggplant, tobacco, tomatoes, potatoes
Nuts–all kinds
Oatmeal
Onion
Pork
Rice
Seeds
Strawberries
Tea
Wheat
Yeast

Foods Allowed
(omit known allergens)

Grains: barley, buckwheat, millet, rye

Herbs: basil, bayleaf, dill, parsley, sage, thyme

Thickeners: arrowroot, tapioca

Fruits: apricot, avocado, rhubarb, blueberries, boysenberries, blackberries, figs, grapes, kiwi, mango, nectarine, olives, papaya, peach, persimmon, pear, pineapple, plums, pomegranate, raspberries

Dried fruits: currants, dates, figs, pineapple, prunes, raisins

Vegetables: artichoke, asparagus, avocado, beets, broccoli, brussels sprouts, cabbage, cantaloupe, carrots, cauliflower, celery, collards, cucumber, honeydew, kale, okra, rutabaga, pumpkin, spinach, squash (acorn, butternut, hubbard, summer, zucchini) sweet potatoes, Swiss chard, turnips, watermelon

120

exercise

A Basketful of Benefits

Exercise was shown to decrease a substance resembling digitalis, which is produced by the body. This substance is manufactured under stress but **reduced with exercise**. It increases the strength and quantity of blood pumped with each beat of the heart. A reduction in this digitalis-like substance may be part of the mechanism that lowers blood pressure with moderate exercise.[111] Exercise is particularly helpful for hypertensive adolescents.[112]

Apart from diet changes, no measure we recommend has so many good effects as physical exercise. Not only does it help the **blood pressure**, it gives **resistance to cancer**, it enhances the **immune system**, **lifts a gloom** from the spirits, **strengthens the bones** and gives many other benefits. You may have many questions like the following: Should I exercise half an hour, three times a week? Should I do easy activities like gardening and walking? Do I need to do all of one day's exercise at one time or can I break it up into segments? Which is most important for health, intensity, duration or frequency of exercise?

Here is good news! **Heavy exercise is not essential** and for some people it may be detrimental, and an added form

122 of stress. Almost any amount of regular mild exercise yields health benefits. You will get approximately 25% lower risk of early death with mild exercise (a stroll around the park) for 20 minutes, four or five times a week; 38% lower risk at 40 minutes, and 50% lower risk if you have an hour or two daily of vigorous, but not violent exercise.[113]

It is not necessary to do all your exercise at one time. Three, 10 minute periods are as effective as one 30-minute stretch. Exercise for at least three days a week is a must and daily exercise is the most helpful.

In most cases exercise has a beneficial effect on the blood pressure. But some normal people experience a transient blood pressure elevation while engaging in heavy exercise. These people are more likely to develop hypertension within six years of beginning a heavy exercise program, as compared to controls who have a normal response to blood pressure with exercise.[114] The key to a proper response is more mild exercise. Describe your workout as moderate or vigorous, but not violent.

How can you tell if you are overtraining? The "no pain, no gain" philosophy can hurt you if you take it too seriously. If you are beginning to have excessive fatigue and declining performance ability you may be overdoing the exercise. Other signs of overtraining are elevation of LDH (lactic dehydrogenase) level in your blood, as determined by a blood test, persistent soreness or tenderness of muscles, a feeling of incomplete recovery between exercise periods, decreased appetite, weight loss, a change in mood or depression, sleep disturbance, an increased susceptibility to infections, increased (or decreased) resting heart rate, anemia, decreased strength and/or hypertension.[115]

While exercising, it is important to wear clothing that protects the extremities from even slight chilling. Blood pressure is very reactive to chilling in some people. The influence of chilling on blood vessels during exercise may be the factor causing the rise in blood pressure in some people following exercise. Many runners and other exercise enthusiasts, start their activities dressed too lightly in cool weather, because they know they will eventually heat up with exertion. This is not a good practice. Ideally, the extremities should be warmly protected in cool weather to reduce the possibility of chilling, and *lightly covered in summer* so that after sweating if a draft blows on the limbs chilling will not result. Chilling pushes the blood disproportionately to the trunk and head causing strain on the heart and arteries. People who die during or just after heavy exercise have usually been dressed in scant clothing which **promotes chilling of the extremities** and overheating of the trunk, even in summer. The great contrast in blood temperature may trigger a fatal heart rhythm disturbance.

The **benefits of exercise** as a treatment for hypertension begin immediately and will have after–exercise advantages even before a state of physical fitness is attained. In contrast, **weight reduction** takes time and **alcohol cessation** requires a recovery and healing period. **Salt and fat reduction**, and a **vegan diet** high in essential minerals, also require time for learning a new way of preparing and enjoying food.

Relaxation techniques require training, but exercise will bring some positive results in minutes.

Nevertheless, certain benefits of exercise do take time, and an exercise program should build up gradually, especially if intensive exercise is the goal.[117]

Weight loss and increased physical exercise can both help the body use insulin more efficiently, which is a big factor in helping hypertension.[118] (See Chapter Three on the relationship of insulin to hypertension.)

One type of exercising has to do with breathing. Breathing with the diaphragm from the abdomen rather than from the upper chest allows the lungs to inflate more extensively and to resist disease better. This also has the good side effect

124 of lowering blood pressure and slowing the heart rate.

Training for abdominal breathing and practicing good posture will both tend to inflate the lungs more and reduce the blood pressure. Instructions on abdominal breathing follow.

How to do abdominal breathing:

1. *Lie on a firm surface* and place a book or one hand on your abdomen.
2. *Concentrate on breathing from your abdomen* instead of from your chest.
3. *Watch* the upward and downward movement of the book or your hand. See how high you can make the book rise up.
4. *Practice abdominal breathing* when you stand up straight.
5. *Make certain you breathe deeply* from the abdomen several times a day. A helpful way to remember to breathe deeply is to decide that each time you pass through a door–car door, room door, house door, etc.– you will take a deep breath.

Begin an exercise program today. Decide what you want and are able to do. Start with something you are certain will not harm you. We suggest walking, gardening, washing the walls of your home a section at a time--your imagination and tastes are the deciding factors--just be careful to start well within your capabilities. Do not rush or push yourself; you could strain or sprain muscles, ligaments or tendons, which will temporarily end your exercise program in a painful way.

Isometric exercises are quite helpful for reducing blood pressure. Running in place and trampoline workouts are useful also, as long as they are not done to the point of being stressful.[119]

weight control program

program guidelines

The following guidelines are for planning a program of weight loss and weight control. By observing these suggestions, the set points will soon be brought down, not only for weight, but also for your blood pressure, your blood sugar, triglycerides, uric acid and cholesterol. This program will encourage normal functioning of the liver, kidneys, heart and arteries.

Cut out all free fats completely. This includes butter, margarine, mayonnaise, fried foods, cooking fats, salad oils, peanut butter and all other nut and seed butters. Flavor is the only reason to add free fats to food and by deleting them from your diet you will not suffer any nutritional deficiency. You will get sufficient essential fatty acids from grains, legumes, nuts, seeds, fruit and vegetables.

Become a total vegetarian. When the Lord made food, he designed certain foods to be produced by animals, as milk for the growth of baby animals. Milk and its byproducts of cheese, butterfat, cottage cheese, cream cheese, yogurt and buttermilk, if fed to young animals, will make them grow.

126

Even the processed fat-free milk byproducts will add weight and mass to young animals because of the growth factor in the protein. If an animal is full-grown and continues to use milk and milk products, it will no longer grow taller or develop a bigger skeletal structure, instead it may grow fat. These products cause growth in human beings also, and most susceptible adults who continue to use milk products will grow fat. Since these foods were not formulated for the adult human body by the Designer, they cause many malfunctions in our body machinery.

Human beings are the only animals who continue to use milk after the age of weaning. Yet, we have greater capabilities to provide an adequate diet. In childhood and youth, the use of all animal products makes us grow quickly and appear to be strong, healthy and robust. But, animal products, plus the intake of our type of diet, with its excessive load of high calories during the younger years, predispose us to many illnesses such as allergies, colds, sore throats, earaches and digestive complaints. They promote early maturation in young children and early puberty with its emotional turbulence–depression, anger, generation gap, unwed sex and juvenile delinquency.[122] As we grow older, these products cause us to become fat and the additional damage caused by them becomes expressed as hypertension, overweight, diabetes, cancer, arthritis or heart disease. No animal product–meat, milk, eggs or cheese–is essential for good nutrition. While animal products contain vital nutrients, all of these nutrients can be obtained in many other types of foods, the same foods the animals eat to get the nutrients.

Eat nothing after three in the afternoon. The metabolism changes at about that time and food taken after 3:00 p.m. makes the set point for weight go up. Drinking herb teas as desired is permissible after three. If you need to be sociable in a group, pour yourself a cup of herbal tea and sip it while enjoying the company of your friends. Carry tea bags with you for emergency use. Never eat a morsel, not even a bite of celery, between meals or after 3:00 p.m.

127

The more raw foods you eat, the better it will be for weight loss. If you are overweight or your blood pressure is quite high, try going for a period of 30 days in which you eat nothing but raw foods. An article published in *Southern Medical Journal* a few years ago reported that not only does weight drop after six months on an all raw diet, but the blood pressure does also.

It is necessary for some people with a delicate stomach, to go through a transition phase before attempting to eat a totally raw food diet. The system is mainly accustomed to digesting cooked foods, and a sudden change to all raw foods could cause minor to severe digestive problems for some people. Slowly increase the quantity of raw foods you are now eating. If your breakfast menu is cereal with canned fruit and milk, add several raw fruits and omit the canned fruit. If your dinner menu is cooked grains, beans and vegetables, try eating the vegetables raw. If you believe yourself to be one of these sensitive people, give yourself about one month to gradually work into a raw food diet. Purchase a raw food recipe book at your local health food store.

Some people will experience digestive problems with raw food, even if they have faithfully followed a transition diet. This is attributed to individual digestive strengths and weaknesses and the physical condition in general. If you notice bloating, constipation or diarrhea, try making raw fruit or vegetable juices with a juicer. Commercial juices will give less benefit. They are no longer fresh and have lost many of their nutrients during shipping and storage. Juices should be taken at the beginning of meals and sipped slowly to mix thoroughly with saliva. Serve fruit juice before a fruit meal and vegetable juice before a vegetable meal. You can also make fruit or vegetable purees in a blender. A vegetable puree can be heated slightly and enjoyed as a thick, warm broth. By using juices and purees, you will still obtain the benefits of raw foods but you will experience less or no digestive upsets.

Breakfast can be fruit in any form—dried, frozen or fresh—with up to 1 tablespoon of nuts or seeds. For lunch try any kind of vegetables in the quantity you desire, along with corn on the cob or whole kernel corn. Limit the variety of foods to no more than four. If you limit the varieties to two or three, that is even better. Some examples of delicious, well-balanced raw lunches are as follows: A large bed of crisp shredded cabbage, finely grated rutabaga, carrot juice with the pulp mixed back in (not the juice alone) and 1/4 to 1/3 cup of shredded unsweetened coconut. Eat this with freshly thawed whole kernel corn in any desired quantity.

Green peas, fresh or frozen or any frozen vegetables (small raw okra is especially healthful), freshly juiced carrots or beets with the pulp added back to the juice and raw sunflower seeds if desired, make a delightful salad. (For a very different texture and flavor, try soaking the sunflower seeds 24-36 hours in water.) Squeeze a few drops of lemon juice on the salad and a sprinkle of dry or fresh mint leaves or sweet basil. This salad would constitute your entire meal.

A fruit salad can be made with apples, oranges and sunflower seeds. You may substitute any other kind of raw seeds or nuts. Certain nuts have more fat than others, and it may, for some, be necessary to severely cut down on the fattier ones. The following nuts and seeds are listed from high fat to low fat content: cashews, pecans, macadamias, walnuts, almonds, coconuts, pistachio, and chestnuts; and sesame, flax, sunflower, and pumpkin seed.

Immediately after meals take some exercise out-of-doors for about 25 minutes. It should not be strenuous, so close

to a meal, but should be moderate or even brisk. Walking, 129
yard work, bicycling (level or downhill), etc., are all good
after-meal exercises. Be sure not to exercise to the point
that you hinder digestion, especially during the first five to
ten minutes after eating.

The smaller the variety of food eaten at one meal, the lower the set point for weight. More weight will be gained from a 600 calorie meal containing ten different dishes made from complex recipes, than a 600 calorie meal containing only two or three simple dishes plus bread and spread. The smaller variety is also beneficial for digestion.

130

herbs, hydrotherapy and nutrient supplements

herbs

Herbs have been used for centuries in the treatment of every human ill. Before 1940 American physicians used many tinctures and teas from herbs. Although they are only beginning to be rediscovered by conventional medicine, herbs are an effective yet harmless therapy when used properly. Unlike drugs for hypertension which almost universally cause serious side effects and sometimes death, herbs generally cause no disturbance, and their proper use will certainly not lead to further illness or death. Furthermore, they are quite effective.

Forms Available. Herbs are most easily used in teas, tinctures, tablets and capsules. Some herbs are available in ointment form, and are more effective when applied to the skin. While herbs are generally best absorbed from the intestinal tract as teas, and are less expensive, the tablets and capsules are more convenient.

132

Diuretic Herbs. Useful teas for lowering blood pressure are the diuretic herbs—watermelon seed, dandelion, cornsilk, buchu, uva ursi and others. You can save seeds from watermelons or buy the seed in a health food store, not a seed store, as they may have been treated with a pesticide. If you have seeds from your own watermelons, rinse and dry them, or for immediate use, prepare tea from fresh seed. Seeds from a store will be already dried. Grind one tablespoon of the seeds in a blender or seed mill. Boil one cup of water, turn heat off, and stir in the ground seeds. Steep 15-30 minutes, strain and drink one to two cups, four times per day. Teas can be made by the quart if desired, but they should be made fresh daily.[123]

Anti-Hypertensive Herbs. Hawthorn berry and black cohosh are also excellent teas for reducing blood pressure. Boil one quart of water and turn heat down to a gentle simmer. Stir in one to three tablespoons of ground hawthorn berry and one-half to three teaspoons of black cohosh. Black cohosh overdosage is recognized by a headache; so, start with about one-half teaspoon and build up by increasing one-half teaspoon per day up to three teaspoons if you are able. If you get a headache, drop down to the quantity which will not cause a headache. Simmer for 20 minutes. Strain and drink the entire quantity in one day. This tea must be made fresh daily in order to be effective.

An extract of *Coleus forskohlii* called *forskolin*, may be very useful. It is a stimulator of cyclic AMP in the blood vessel wall, which causes relaxation of smooth muscle and lowering of blood pressure. Two capsules three or four times a day should be taken.

Garlic is a time-honored remedy for hypertension. It is very beneficial when used in a combined program with other herbal products and changes in lifestyle. We have not had remarkable reduction in blood pressure with garlic alone, perhaps because we have not used large enough quantities. It may require several heads of garlic daily, perhaps one or two at each meal, to effect significant blood pressure reductions.

We had a case of a 64 year old woman who had tried garlic extract capsules and magnesium aspartate for three months, along with dietary and lifestyle changes, and had only reduced her blood pressure from around 155/84 to around 140/80. Then she got a very severe case of flu, and in order to try to stay on her job began eating a very light diet and taking two globes (10-12 cloves each) of fresh garlic three times a day, along with the same dosage of garlic capsules and magnesium aspartate as before. She dropped her blood pressure in two days to 128/78. Furthermore, when we have used the concentrated forms of garlic such as Kyolic liquid (the Japanese "cold- aged" garlic) in a large dosage of one to three teaspoons three times a day, we have had better results than with the dried garlic in capsules. Kitchen garlic powder or garlic salt may be completely ineffective, as the garlic may be several years old before it gets to your home.

Herbs to Slow Heart Rate. Mistletoe has been reported to slow the heart rate and to lower blood pressure. Put two teaspoons of the leaves in two cups of boiling water, set aside to steep for 10 minutes. Take one cup in the morning and one at night. Make up fresh every day.

Lily of the valley is also very good to slow the pulse rate. Its active ingredient is a digitaloid, plus a slight diuretic effect. Onset of action on the heart is within 30 minutes. Its elimination begins rapidly so that there is no accumulation in the body of the herb. Paradoxically, not only does lily of the valley slow the rapid heart, but in the form of congestive heart failure which has a slow heartbeat, lily of the valley is very good to use to relieve the heart failure. While it is not as good as foxglove (digitalis) in severe cases, it can be very helpful for milder forms. Use one tablespoon of the herb in one quart of boiling water. Set off the fire to steep for 20 minutes. Many herbalists consider lily of the valley to be toxic,

134 apparently due to its digitalis-like effect. In our experience we have not found it to be so. However, it should probably not be used if the patient is taking a digitalis preparation, and the dosage above should not be exceeded. Other herbs may be added at the time lily of the valley is put in.

Anticlotting Herbs. Motherwort has an anticlotting effect and can be useful to help prevent clotting within the blood vessels. This herb also has a good effect to normalize the rhythm of the heart. It may be used in atrial fibrillation, palpitations and tachycardia. Use two tablespoons of the chopped plant in a quart of gently simmering water for 20 minutes. Drink the quart throughout the day. May be mixed with other herbs, as can all the herbs in this section.

Skullcap was demonstrated in two Japanese studies to increase levels of HDL, the "good cholesterol." This effect has a beneficial effect on the characteristics of blood, which directly affects the flow properties of blood and indirectly the blood pressure. Since skullcap also has tranquilizing actions, it is a good choice for tense persons who have high blood pressure. Make the tea in the same way as for lily of the valley.

Garlic also has very potent anticlotting factors. It may be used as described above, and should be very helpful as it has more than one benefit for the person who has high blood pressure.

Herbs to Use With Caution. People with hypertension should use care if they take Ginseng, Kelp, Kola, St. John's Wort, Licorice or Ephedra as these have been reported occasionally to cause an elevation in blood pressure for some people. Large doses of Juniper taken longer than six weeks can raise blood pressure. Licorice in large quantities can cause low potassium and hypertension and mimic an adrenal disease called aldosteronism. Glycyrrhizic acid is the component in Licorice which interferes with hormone and mineral balance if glycyrrhiza is taken in large quantities and too frequently. Too much licorice will also cause sodium to be retained and potassium to be lost. Weight then goes up because of fluid retention.[124] People who took one-half cup (eight tablespoons) of the Licorice powder daily for eight weeks had an increase in body weight of nearly four pounds, presumably from fluid retention.

hydrotherapy

A hot foot bath lowers the blood pressure from 2-20 points.[125] It works by a reflexive involuntary response. As the hot water causes the blood vessels in the foot to expand, blood is drawn away from vessels in the trunk, and into dilated vessels far from the heart.

As the blood redistributes throughout the body, the tension at any one point is greatly reduced. The foot bath functions by breaking up the congestion and constriction of blood vessels in the trunk and freeing the blood to flow easily through the entire body.

A 20-90 minute neutral (95-100 degrees) or hot (100-110 degrees) bath will always lower acutely elevated blood pressure. Caution should be used not to step into the water when it is very hot. Aside from the fact that it can scald the skin, the blood pressure can go up within the first 20-60 seconds because of the extreme change in skin temperature. If the blood pressure is already very high, the level could conceivably rise very high in the first minute. During the first minute, sit in the slightly warm bath, then run in more hot water if desired; breathe deeply and the blood pressure should fall in about three to five minutes. Within 10-15 minutes it should drop lower than before the application of heat, sometimes dramatically so. If the bath water is hot enough, or the bath is continued for long enough, the mouth temperature will begin to rise and the pulse rate will also rise, about 10 beats

136 per degree of temperature elevation. If the mouth temperature does not rise too high, the bath can be continued for several hours, as long as the blood pressure stays down. Check blood pressure every 20 minutes.

Fomentations (hot compresses or hot wet towels) can also be used to bring blood pressure down. One method is to lie on a long heating pad — one which covers most of the spine. Or, cover the bed with plastic, put hot wet towels lengthwise down the bed with one or two dry towels on top. Lie down on the hot towels. Place a second hot towel on the front of the trunk, covered with plenty of dry towels to keep the heat in. The feet should be put in very warm water. Keep the towels hot and the foot bath warm for 20-90 minutes or more. For insulin dependent diabetics, your physician has already instructed you not to use hot water on your feet. Follow this instruction because your feet are more susceptible to blistering. All diabetics should use caution with hot water.

supplements

Magnesium is quite useful for assisting blood pressure control, therefore should probably be a part of every regimen for the usual case of non–complicated, high blood pressure, or so-called essential hypertension.

It is quite a safe treatment and many decades have found it as a trusted home remedy for a variety of ills. For more than half a century we have treated women who have certain types of toxemia of pregnancy with magnesium sulfate. Some have believed this baffling disease, characterized by rising blood pressure, protein in the urine and swelling of the entire body with sometimes enormous weight gain due to retained tissue fluid, was caused by magnesium deficiency brought on by the increased need for extra nutrients during pregnancy. This problem has not been clarified as yet, but women nowadays get far less toxemia than formerly, possibly due to improved nutrition with greater magnesium content of the diet.

A number of well-done studies have recently shown magnesium to be deficient in virtually every case of hypertension. It is a smooth muscle relaxer, helping to open up the constricted arterioles (the smallest of arteries). A simple supplement is Epsom salts (magnesium sulfate), one teaspoon on the back of the tongue or in a small glass of water two or three times a day. The rare person may experience diarrhea from this small dose, in which case switch to capsules containing other magnesium salts (chloride, citrate, or aspartate). Magnesium is best absorbed if taken with or very close to a meal.

L-arginine is an amino acid, the major precursor in the body for nitric oxide. Nitric oxide has been found to be generated on demand by the endothelium (lining cells) of arterioles, and relaxes smooth muscle. It was formerly called "endothelium relaxing factor." L-arginine, given in a dosage of 1000 milligrams four times daily on an empty stomach, may be very useful in blood pressure control.

Although it is apparently innocuous, we do not have longterm studies on prolonged use of L-arginine. Therefore, we suggest it only be used for about a month at a time, then omit for at least two weeks to see if the blood pressure can be maintained without it.

Some of the highest food sources of arginine are peanuts, walnuts, pecans, rolled oats, spaghetti, shredded wheat, limas, kidney beans and peas.

138

what other people did to get well

case histories

Emotions and High Blood Pressure
The relationship of hidden emotions to high blood pressure is shown by the following two stories.

Jane. We were counseling a woman who was having severe stress in her marriage. Jane suppressed her feelings and denied the existence of any problems. Although prior to her marriage she had been advised not to marry Roger, she ignored the advice and proceeded with the marriage. After 15 years her marriage had become a constant and nearly intolerable difficulty. Her pulse rate would rise to 160 during a short walk even though she was physically fit. Her blood pressure also rose from approximately 102/58 to around 128/85. Despite a good Health Recovery Program, these physical signs continued for months and were an enigma to her physicians. She was faithful to eliminate all salt and fat from her diet and she became a total vegetarian. Each day she carried out a suitable exercise workout, and her weight was ideal.

Within a few months, her marital problems erupted to the surface. Three months after admitting her true feelings about her husband and marriage and getting appropriate counseling, her heart rate and blood pressure began to return to normal.

Allie Mae. Another patient was named Allie Mae Thomas. Her work as a solitary travel agent often kept her up late into the night. When we began treating her for high blood pressure, her readings were approximately 190/98. With diet, herb teas, and regularity in sleep times, meal times and exercise, she finally had consistent levels of about 130/82.

One night a family member, who was a nurse, took her blood pressure reading just as she lay down to sleep. The reading was 125/76. Her relative then began a ten minute footrub which was known to relax Allie Mae and reduce her blood pressure. During the footrub, the nurse began relating to Allie Mae a bit of disturbing family gossip. After about ten minutes of the unpleasant gossip Allie Mae's blood pressure was up to 167/88. It is reasonable to assume, based on findings such as this, that some people have sustained high blood pressure because of living in a situation of unresolved trial.

Nobody needs to carry a heavy weight of worry. Through prayer and study of the Scriptures you can transfer your troubles to our Savior who has provided for all our needs. Faith is trusting God; believing that He loves us and knows best what is for our good. Thus instead of our own will, it leads us to choose His will. Instead of our ignorance, it accepts His wisdom; instead of our weakness, His strength; instead of our sinfulness, His righteousness.

Overweight and High Insulin

We had a 19-year-old patient at the health center at Uchee Pines with high blood pressure. He was the son of a physician, and had blood pressure readings above 200/110. The ideal at his age should be well below 120/80. He was 5'8" and weighed somewhat over 200 pounds, more than 50 pounds overweight, and told us he was always hungry, even immediately after a meal (a good sign of high blood insulin). His blood insulin level was borderline high even when he was fasting; but two hours after he ate, it was quite elevated. Normal is under 30--his level was 95, even though his blood sugar was normal! We started his program with a five day fast followed by the Health Recovery Program (See Chapter Nine). The diet along with a restricted salt intake and an exercise program were sufficient to bring his blood pressure down quickly. He started losing weight and feeling good. He never once complained of hunger after the fast because his insulin levels went down and his appetite had become so regulated, that with a proper diet, he was quite satisfied with what he ate.

It is important to recognize the fact, taught by this case, that insulin is a potent stimulant of the appetite. This is one reason people who are going to develop diabetes may have such a difficult time controlling the appetite. If they would tough it out for a few weeks with reduced calories in the diet, the insulin levels would fall, the appetite would lose its stimulus from insulin overproduction and the weight could be kept in much better control. Where most people with constantly increasing weight make their big mistake is by indulging appetite occasionally as a treat to themselves. **It is no treat to eat incorrectly.** One must always pay with days of struggle with the appetite. The difficulty with this kind of occasional "vacation" from a good diet is that even this rare indiscretion causes the pancreas to react with overproduction of insulin for days. By then, it is time for another "vacation" and the appetite struggle never ceases. The poor person is always on the battle field.

142

An Overweight Nurse

BS. This was a 51 year old black female, a geriatric nurse from Bermuda. She was 5'2" tall and weighed 242 pounds. She had a long family history of hypertension. Her blood pressure while taking both Nifedipine and Atenolol was 140/96 on arrival, but fell to 114/70 after three weeks even though she then took no medication. She lost 14 pounds during her three weeks on a total vegetarian, salt–free diet, down to 228 pounds. She was also treated with massage three times weekly, several herbal teas, two Kyolic capsules three times a day, and magnesium sulfate, one teaspoonful twice a day. She received Russian steam baths seven times during the three weeks. Her exercise was to her own tolerance, and upon arrival was less than two blocks a day, but by the time she had spent three weeks in our patient program, she could walk almost two miles. Two days each week she fasted, Tuesday and Friday. We have found that fasting greatly improves the person's blood pressure and those who have diabetes are always much improved.

How Herbs get a Bad Name

Mr. CS. The following report from a medical journal is an illustration of how natural remedies and lifestyle changes get a bad name. Mr. CS, a 61 year old black man from Detroit, had a blood pressure around 160/98. He was treated with a number of medications by an internist at Ford Hospital. All the medicines they gave him had unpleasant side effects, and he refused to try others. He then began on his own to take garlic. For six months he took garlic and dropped his blood pressure to around 130-140 over 80-85. He probably took at least the equivalent of ten cloves or one bulb with each meal (10-15 capsules of aged garlic) in order to get such a good response.

He returned to his doctor and told him what he had done. The doctor then wanted to try a scientific study on him. He stopped the garlic for a week (called a washout period) then began treatment with three pairs of garlic-smelling placebos or garlic twice a day for three weeks each. During the week he was off garlic his blood pressure rose to an average of 148.9/89.6. Then he was given an insignificant quantity of dried garlic–1/2gm, which is about 1/10th teaspoon. The quantity of garlic given the man was equivalent to fresh garlic of 1.25 gm. or 1/5 teaspoon. But the dried, powdered kitchen variety was used, a kind we rarely use because of the great variation in potency from one batch to another. We would have given doses 20-40 times as high, and not twice a day, but three or four times a day until the blood pressure was in a satisfactory range. With the kitchen garlic powder, there is no assurance of the freshness of the garlic. If it is not less than six months old, there can be quite a reduction in the active ingredient. On the tiny dose his blood pressure only fell from 148.9/89.6 to 146.9/87.2. We marvel that it fell any. The case was reported in a medical journal to illustrate the lack of response to be expected from garlic, but I think the doctor doing the experiment at Henry Ford Hospital in Detroit did not know how to design a good experiment with garlic, and did not counsel with those who had had experience with this herb.[134] Furthermore, those employed to do a review of the article and criticize the investigator's work did not know enough about his method and the matter they were reviewing to act as experts in this issue. The Journal should have employed an herbalist acquainted with treatment of patients with garlic to review the work and give counsel.

Hypertension for 13 Years
MS. This 76-year-old white female from Pennsylvania came to the Lifestyle Center with obesity (184 pounds), insomnia, hypertension, and vertigo which developed after a fall one year before. She was of Cuban-American extraction and had lived most of the last 40 years in the United States.

144 She weighed 185 pounds when she arrived and had a blood pressure of 160/95. She was treated with daily massage, fomentations to the chest, abdomen, and back three times a week with exercise to her tolerance considering her age and overweight condition, and with a salt-free vegetarian diet. She was given two tablespoons of freshly ground flaxseed with each meal. She also took a number of herbal teas including buchu and uva ursi (diuretic teas), valerian and wood betony (sedative teas), and ginkgo (two capsules three times daily) for her circulation and to open up blood vessels in the internal organs. After three weeks her blood pressure was 145/82, her weight was 172, and she felt much better in every way. Her insomnia was somewhat less and her vertigo was much improved. She had had hypertension for 13 years, most of which time she had taken very toxic pharmaceuticals. She was happy to be off the medications, and very pleased that her blood pressure was actually lower off the medication and on her program than before.

Diabetes and Hypertension

GS. This 62-year-old black female from Atlanta, Georgia was seen at the Lifestyle Center at Uchee Pines because of overweight, diabetes and hypertension. She weighed 212 pounds, had a lot of edema in both feet, judged at four-plus, and her blood pressure was 210/130, even though she was faithfully taking diltiazem. Her diabetes had become complicated with diabetic neuropathy in both legs. She was given a vegan diet (vegetarian without meat, milk, eggs, or cheese) with an emphasis on citrus fruits (especially grapefruit), beans and peas, peanuts and cantaloupe for her diabetic neuropathy, and had magnesium citrate in maximum dosage. She was also given hawthorne berry tea and valerian root for its sedative qualities. By the end of the three week session she was down to 200 pounds and her blood pressure had fallen to 150/78. Her HDL, which was 30 on admission, was 40 by the end of the three week session. Her LDL had been 173, and was down to 133 upon discharge. The triglycerides were 257 on arrival, and 204 on leaving. Her blood sugar with insulin was 206, but fell to 145 without insulin after fasting a day or two per week for three weeks..

Hypertension Beginning in Pregnancy

YS. This 44 year old Jamaican female, 5' 1" tall and weighing 147 pounds, began having elevated blood pressure in the third trimester of her pregnancy in 1986. She tried many different kinds of blood pressure medicines, but all left her with very unpleasant side effects. When she did not take blood pressure medicines she had very severe migraine headaches. Her blood pressure on arrival was 180/110. She was taking Cardura. During the three week session she was weaned down to half the dosage she had been taking upon arrival and her blood pressure had fallen to 140/92. Her weight loss was only seven pounds. She was given a salt free, vegan diet. Other treatments included warm tub baths (98-100 degrees F), Russian steam baths once or twice a week, and daily full body massage. She took two capsules of magnesium citrate three times a day, Kyolic liquid two times a day, and one tablespoon of flax seed oil twice a day. She took hawthorne berry, yarrow, and valerian root teas, one cup three times daily.

Great improvement in 21 Days

AS. This 57-year-old black female from Nassau was only 5'4" tall, yet she weighed 215 pounds. Her blood pressure was 154/90 at the beginning of the patient session. She took Natrilix three times daily upon arrival, but after three weeks she was taking no medicine, but her blood pressure was 150/88, approximately the same as at the beginning of the session with the medication. She took a salt-free vegan diet and daily exercise, several herbal teas and one tablespoon of flaxseed freshly ground with each meal. Her pulse was 84 upon arrival and 72 when she left. Her total cholesterol was 201 when she arrived and had fallen to 158 after three weeks. Her uric acid went from 6.3 to 6.0 in three weeks (ideal is from 2.1 to 5.0). Her HDL which was 24 on arrival (normals from 35-85), had risen to 37. Her LDL at 155 on arrival (less than 110 is ideal) had fallen to 120. Her triglycerides were 211 on arrival and had fallen to 101 when she left.

Familial Hypertension

JS, was a 71-year-old overweight Hispanic female from Illinois. She had diabetes for which she took Glucatrol. She had hypertension and came from a family with a strong history of hypertension, stating that "her whole family was hypertensive." She felt that her own blood pressure was related to stress. She was given a two-meal plan, with one to two days per week of total fasting in which she took nothing but water. She was encouraged to walk as far as she was able to walk, which usually turned out to be up to three miles a day. Her weight upon arrival was 161 and fell to 157 after three weeks. Her triglycerides were 243 on arrival and 141 at the end of the three week session. Her blood sugar level while taking Glucatrol was 161 on arrival and 132 without any medications upon discharge. Her cholesterol was 191 on arrival and 137 at the time she left. Her blood pressure was 150/80 on three hypertensive medications and 150/78 on no medications by the time she had spent three weeks at the Lifestyle Center.

Fatigue and Hypertension

GS, a 32-year-old black female from Nassau, came to our Lifestyle Center complaining of extreme fatigue and an eight-year history of hypertension. She was 5'4" and weighed 155 pounds. Her last pregnancy had to be terminated four to five weeks early with a Cesarean section because of a rising blood pressure and increasing protein in her urine. She was taking Procardia and her blood pressure was 150/105. In three weeks she was entirely off medications, and her blood pressure was 140/88. Her serum iron was 193 (ideal levels from 20-85, although the reference range is usually said to be 40–150, too high for the best of health, as higher levels have been found to be associated with a greater risk of heart attacks, strokes and cancer), and fell to 95. Cholesterol at 184 on arrival fell to 114. Her LDL of 114 fell to 62. Her blood sugar was 92 on arrival and 89 when she left.

Illustration of Failure

RB. A 49-year-old black female came from a northern state. She was a frequent patient at our Lifestyle Center and was treated for a number of things through the years. She had not only hypertension up to 210/110, but overweight (237 pounds). Her case was complicated by sarcoidosis and a cancer of the breast. She had had a hysterectomy.

She was never able to stay on a program. We tried many combinations of diet, herbal teas, nutrient supplements, exercise, and many other kinds of programs. Her intentions were always good, but she was never able to discipline herself sufficiently to become victorious.

After her stroke, she lost weight to 172 pounds and her blood pressure fell on its own to 114/75. This is an illustration of failure to gain the victory over the great American lifestyle. When it becomes entrenched in childhood, it sometimes requires a miracle from heaven or a calamity to deliver one from the damaging lifestyle. There is victory through prayer and a determined effort.

A Georgia Woman

CL. A 64-year-old white female came to us from Georgia. Her blood pressure on arrival was 180/90, and she was treated with one tablespoon of flaxseed oil twice a day for its antiinflammatory qualities, a dish of prunes daily for their

148 laxative effect, ginkgo biloba tea, one quart every day as a vasodilator, pycnogenol as an antioxidant and general tonic and eight garlic tablets daily for her blood pressure. Her blood pressure was stabilized in the 140 over 80 range during the patient session. Her cholesterol on admission was 234, and 205 at the time she left three weeks later. Her triglycerides were 136 on arrival and 92 three weeks later.

Success with a very simple program

RB. This 63-year-old black male came from Tennessee. He had a diagnosis of borderline hypertension at 144/84, weight of 210 and triglycerides of 299 on arrival. His weight was 210 pounds on arrival and fell to 198 pounds when he was ready to leave at the end of the three week session. His blood pressure had fallen to 108/64. He was treated with one tablespoon of charcoal four times a day for his elevated triglycerides, and with a salt-free vegan diet (and weight loss) as his only treatments for the borderline hypertension. The simple program was very successful in bringing his blood pressure to a very good level.

The Effect of Disturbing News

HD, This 65 year old black female was from Canada, but of Jamaican descent. She had a 30 year history of high blood pressure for which she took Adalat, 60 milligrams daily, Pindalol, .5 milligrams twice a day, Apo-triazide, one per day, and Digoxin, 0.125 milligram daily. She was treated at our clinic with two tablespoons of freshly ground flaxseed with each meal, the juice of chayote (a squash-like vegetable), two to three times a week, no refined sugar, flours, or oils, a neutral tub bath 20-30 minutes twice a day, and a full-body massage three times a week to increase her peripheral circulation. She was given magnesium citrate, two capsules three times a day, hawthorne berry tea, one cup three times a day, and peppermint and rosemary tea with thyme as she needed it for sedation. She was on a salt-free vegan diet. During the three week stay, the patient was able to stop her medications. When she arrived at Uchee Pines, her blood pressure readings averaged around 160/100. After she started taking our treatments and leaving off the medications, her readings averaged 145/80. The very day after she stopped taking the blood pressure medication, she received a call from home which was very disturbing. She was weeping and became discouraged and her blood pressure went up to 215/110. For this she was given a neutral tub bath at 97 degrees and a whole globe of garlic, steamed for 10-12 minutes and served with lemon juice. She received a full body massage and rested for one hour at which time her blood pressure was 150/75.

A diabetic hypertensive from Detroit

KM was a 71-year-old black male from Detroit. His diagnoses upon arrival were overweight, high blood pressure, and diabetes. He was treated with two tablespoons of freshly ground flaxseed with each meal, a salt-free vegan diet and the health recovery program described in this book. He increased his walking so that by two weeks he was walking six to seven miles per day. He began a fast after he had been here for one week and spent five days in the fast and five days gradually breaking his fast. He took one cup of hawthorne berry tea three times a day, two capsules of magnesium citrate three times a day, and herbs for his diabetes—bay leaf, oregano, dandelion, and sage. His blood pressure when he arrived was 190/90, and on leaving 145/62. His glucose readings were 186 and 138 respectively, cholesterol 224 (LDL 123, HDL 26), and 222 (LDL 121 and HDL 28). His triglycerides were 373 and 265 respectively.

15 pounds in three weeks!

AB. We had a 60 year old black female come from the Bahamas with diagnoses on arrival of diabetes, carpal tunnel

150 syndrome, borderline hypertension and intestinal gas. She was treated with pyridoxin (vitamin B-6, 100 milligrams daily), vanadyl sulfate, 15 mg before meals, one tablespoon of flax-seed oil with each meal, and two tablespoons of freshly ground flaxseed with each meal. She was given the health recovery program outlined in this book. Her admission and discharge reports are as follows—glucose 191 and 139; LDL 229 and 166; cholesterol 268 and 205; blood pressure 165/90 and 124/80. She learned the two-meal a day plan very easily and lost from 205 pounds to 190 pounds during three weeks. She said her husband would be most surprised that she did not eat suppers anymore since they had always been her favorite meal of the day. Now she said breakfast would become her favorite meal.

Severely abnormal HDL and hemoglobin

JB. This was a 69 year old black male from Maryland. When he arrived at the Lifestyle Center his diagnoses were overweight (222 pounds), hypertension (120/90 while on three blood pressure medications), arteriosclerotic heart disease and polycythemia vera (too many red blood cells). He was taking a medication to make his cholesterol come down and on admission his cholesterol was 171. He stopped taking the medication while at Uchee Pines Lifestyle Center, and his cholesterol went to 191. We sometimes see the cholesterol go up in people who already have severe hardening of the arteries, and it seems that in these individuals, a reabsorption of cholesterol from the arteries and tissues is the factor causing the blood cholesterol to stay up. His HDL, the good cholesterol, went up from 21 (severely depressed) to 34, only slightly depressed. His triglycerides were 234 on arrival and 194 when he left three weeks later. He fasted three days each week, Monday, Wednesday, and Friday, and had a unit of blood withdrawn for his polycythemia which brought his hemoglobin from 16.8 to 14.9 at the time he left.

His treatments included a salt-free vegan diet, one tablespoon of flaxseed freshly ground with each of two meals, two ginkgo capsules three times a day, three magnesium citrate capsules three times a day for his blood pressure, as well as two capsules of Kyolic three times a day for blood pressure, and five to six steamed cloves of garlic with each lunch meal. He lost 24 pounds during the three weeks. He felt that his most important single victory while at Uchee Pines was learning not to overeat and taking only two meals per day. He said that for years he had known that he overate, but that the quality of his appetite was such that he was never able to control it. He stated that he was now a new man and hoped to be able to help his entire church to gain the victory over appetite.

152

hypertension drugs and complications

The American Association of Retired Persons (AARP) carried the following sad statement in their *News Bulletin* in April, 1989: "Tens of thousands of older people are living in an inhuman and needless stupor induced by misuse or over-use of prescription drugs, medical experts told reporters last month..."

Speaker after speaker said that over-drugging is a major problem for older people. The report, written by Richard P. Kusserow, inspector general of the Department of Health and Human Services, cited a series of systematic weaknesses throughout the drug delivery system. Among them were mis-diagnoses by doctors, faulty prescriptions and improper use of drugs by patients.

"Another problem is that patients are sometimes put on four prescription medicines to control high blood pressure when one would do....The experts noted that 51% of deaths from drugs in the United States involve people 60 or older, even though these older Americans account for only 17% of the population." What a statement!

More doctors today are beginning to question the growing popularity of drugs to treat high blood pressure. It is now

154 recognized that many of these drugs increase risks of heart attacks, cancers, altered metabolism in the liver, kidneys, immune and nervous systems (affecting emotions, behavior and muscle function).

Scientists from the National Institutes of Health released the results in September 1982[14] of a decade-long, nationwide study of 13,000 men. This study revealed an unexpectedly high death rate in those treated with blood pressure drugs. Men with abnormal EKG readings who were treated with drugs had a 65% higher rate of mortality than those in a control group who did not receive drugs.

In 1982, Dr. Norman Caplan of the University of Texas, pointed out that the already high level of drug use for hypertension has risen 10-20% in the last five years. This had occurred at a time researchers were publishing reports on studies showing the effectiveness of non-drug treatments for hypertension. He went on to say, "We are unnecessarily treating with drugs a rather large percentage of the hypertensive population." (He believed that to be about 20 million of the 60 million Americans now labeled as having high blood pressure.)[15, 16, 17]

Diuretics

Diuretics May Cause High Cholesterol

A study reported in the *Journal of the American Medical Association* in June 1988, revealed abnormal blood cholesterol and high triglycerides in those patients who were taking diuretics and beta blockers. The abnormal cholesterol was made up of low levels of good cholesterol (HDL) and high levels of bad cholesterol (LDL). Dr. Roger Williams of the University of Utah said the abnormal blood fats were probably more dangerous than high blood pressure.

In 1990 the *New York Times* carried a front page article

with the following headline: "New Study Says Diuretics Raise Heart Attack Risks." About 200 other newspapers picked up the *Times* article. The Associated Press carried a separate report and warned their readers, "Patients taking diuretics...were urged to ask their doctors about a new study showing that these drugs may increase the risk of a heart attack." The report which the *Times* and the AP are referring to is that by Pollare, T. and co-workers, published in the *New England Journal of Medicine.* [18]

Diuretics Escalate Kidney Cancer Risk in Men

With the increasing length of time patients use diuretics and the increase of diuretic use in general, there is an escalating risk of renal cell cancer (kidney), particularly in men.[19]

Another risk with diuretics, as well as with other drugs, is that drugs taken before pregnancy can cause abnormalities in the structure of the unborn child. If we are discovering such profound changes in the unborn, it is just as reasonable to believe that these same "teratogenic" drugs (those causing severe abnormal growth alterations) can cause disorders in functions of the adult body such as the delicate functioning of the liver, spleen, pancreas, bone marrow, etc., as it is to believe they can cause structural changes in the unborn child. This association was discovered by keeping records of all the hormonal drugs, the dietary recommendations and other measures taken by a group of women during pregnancy. The information from the maternal records, was then correlated with the appearance of high blood pressure in the offspring.[20]

For the past half century, the retention of sodium has been the rationale for the use of the diuretic drugs for high blood pressure. Beginning with mercurial diuretics in the 1940's, followed by chlorothiazide and hydrochlorothiazide, (Diuril, Hydrodiuril) and more recently, Lasix, have all been the most commonly prescribed drugs to diurese sodium. As mentioned earlier, these diuretics not only do not reduce the risk of having a heart attack, they actually *increase* it, especially when beta blockers such as Inderal, Atenolol, and others that slow the pulse rate are used as well. There is additionally an increased incidence of coronary artery operations for people with hypertension who are treated with diuretics or beta blockers. The reason for this is that both of these classes of drugs have adverse effects by enhancing insulin resistance, of increasing blood cholesterol and triglycerides, and adversely affecting metabolism. This detrimental influence outweighs the beneficial results of lowering the blood pressure.

Treatment of high blood pressure with most drugs causes a paradox. Drugs will markedly decrease the risk of a stroke, congestive heart failure, and kidney failure. But according to 13 studies, in which people were observed over the course of many years to discover what cumulative effects result from the long-term use of blood pressure medications, there is no decrease in the risk of having a heart attack or having coronary heart disease by lowering blood pressure with drugs. Studies in Sweden have shown that people with high blood pressure who have been treated with diuretics or beta blockers for ten years, have a tenfold increased risk of Type II diabetes. Because most of the drugs used to treat high blood pressure have such adverse effects on hyperinsulinism and elevated blood fats, any beneficial effects they may have are negated and the chances of increased risks for early death are greater.

Roughly one-third of all new dialysis patients are people with hypertension. High blood pressure in itself will cause damage to the kidneys.[21] Researchers measured blood levels of a waste protein called creatinine and found that creatinine levels gradually increased the longer a person has hypertension. This rise is evidence of kidney damage. It is plain to see that the treatment of hypertension is beneficial for reasons other than simply lowering the risk of strokes. This treatment, however, is best done without drugs.

According to information from the manufacturers, verapamil, known as Calan, Isoptin, Verelan and Verin, and other drugs for hypertension may cause blurred vision. It is not known whether they produce other eye changes also, such as cataracts.

To determine the effects of prenatal drug exposure, animals have been given hormonal drugs and much salt to test for blood pressure changes in their offspring. High blood pressure at maturity was discovered in animals who had been prenatally subjected to the drugs and salt. The condition of the animals is very similar to the type of hypertension seen in human beings who were congenitally exposed to large amounts of hormones and salt.

Most antihypertensive drugs also cause behavioral side effects that are unacceptable. These can range from mild dizziness to delirium or severe depression, unwanted sedation, sleep disturbance, impairment of sexual functions, inter–reactions with other psycho-active drugs, sleep walking, violent behavior and amnesia. Patients may stay on medication only because the doctor told them they have to, even though their quality of life has been lowered.[22]

A report in the *Archives of Internal Medicine* stated the following conclusions: "Our data indicate that a nonpharmacologic intervention will lower both systolic and diastolic blood pressure levels..."[23]

To lower blood presssure, the researchers "focused on calorie and sodium reduction with increases in moderate levels of physical activity." They suggested less than 1200 calories for women and less than 1500 calories for men per day. Sodium was reduced to 1400 milligrams daily. Physical activity (slow walking) was begun for 120 minutes each week (four 30 minute sessions). The results were very good.

Physiological Treatments are Best
Most people who are taking antihypertensive drugs can

158 stop their medications completely if they will lose weight and reduce their salt intake. You can start to do this on your own. Keep taking your drugs until you are well into the program; then taper them off, rather than suddenly dropping them. Some persons will have a jump in blood pressure if they simply drop their medicines.

Begin with a salt and weight reduction program, including exercise, while continuing to take your medication and visiting your doctor. Your blood pressure should be checked several times per week, preferably at home with your own equipment. You may wish to ask your doctor's office nurse to monitor you as you proceed with your new program. You will start to observe a fall in blood pressure. Your medication will then need to be reduced rapidly enough to keep you from getting hypotension — levels below 100/70 (higher levels may be desirable for older people; your doctor can give you a safe level). [24, 25]

When you are following an improved lifestyle routine and are no longer taking blood pressure medication, your blood pressure will not fall too low if you use only the suggested natural treatments. But with synthetic, laboratory created medicines, your blood pressure is liable to fall to dangerous lows or climb to alarming heights.

Dr. Thomas Pickering, Professor of Medicine at the New York Hospital-Cornell Medical Center, presents the fact that there has not been shown much, if any, benefit of drug therapy for white women before menopause. Yet these drugs have potentially serious side effects.[26] Dr. Pickering says you are more likely to be prescribed drugs in America, than in Europe, for the same level of blood pressure. Yet mortality rates from cardiovascular disease are lower in Europe than in the United States.

Antihypertensive Drugs
The following list, taken from the 1997 edition of *The*

Physicians' Desk Reference (The *PDR*) unless otherwise indicated, includes the most commonly prescribed drugs for blood pressure. Side effects of these drugs are also included. You can read the *PDR* at a library. As we study the side effects of drugs, and recognize the many natural and non-harmful remedies for high blood pressure, it becomes difficult to understand why drugs are prescribed as initial treatment for hypertension when so many of them take serious chances with the patient's health. Most drugs of this class have a deleterious effect on cholesterol and triglycerides, except for the ACE inhibitors, the alpha antagonists and the calcium channel blockers.[27] Yet, these last named drugs have still other side effects, as shown below:

Calcium Channel Blockers--Calcium ion inhibitor, page 210 of 1994 *PDR*

Description
Calcium antagonists which inhibit the transfer of calcium ions into cardiac muscle and smooth muscle. The contraction of cardiac muscle and the smooth muscles of blood vessels are dependent upon the movement of calcium into these cells through specific channels.

Conventional Prescription Names
Adalat, Calan, Cardede, Cardizem, DynaCirc, Isoptin, Nimotop, Plendil, Procardia, Vascor

Warnings
Excessively low blood pressure, increased urinary frequency, duration and severity of angina or acute heart attacks and congestive heart failure are all more likely to occur. (!)

Adverse Reactions
•Central Nervous System: Dizziness, giddiness,

160

lightheadedness, nervousness, blurred vision, difficulty with balance, sleep disturbances, depression, memory loss, paranoia, fatigue
- Heart and Arteries: Peripheral edema, palpitations, syncope, dangerously low heart rate, heart block (AV)
- Respiratory: Nasal and chest congestion, shortness of breath, cough, wheezing
- Gastrointestinal: Nausea, heartburn, diarrhea, constipation, cramps, flatulence, allergic hepatitis
- Systemic: Headache, flushing, weakness
- Musculo-Skeletal: Inflammation, joint stiffness, muscle cramps
- Other: Dermatitis, itching, hives, fever, sweating, chills, sexual difficulties including impotence

Beta-Blocking Agents--page 1032, 1994 PDR

Description
Blocks beta-adrenergic receptors (part of the nerve impulse transmission system), and competes with beta-adrenergic receptor stimulating agents for available receptor sites. When access is blocked to these sites the chronotropic, inotropic and vasodilator responses to beta adrenergic stimulation is decreased proportionately. (This means that the system for sending certain types of nerve impulses all over the body, as well as in the brain, are blocked. Certain types of responses your brain and nerves are designed to make will be obstructed.)

Conventional Prescription Names
Blocadren, Cartrol, Corgard, Corzide, Inderal, Inderide, Kerlone, Levatol, Lopressor, Normozide, Tenoretic, Timolide, Visken

Adverse Reactions

- Central Nervous System: Dizziness, tiredness, depression, headaches, nightmares, insomnia, confusion
- Heart and Arteries: Shortness of the breath, excessively slow heart rate, cold extremities, palpitations, congestive heart failure, peripheral edema, excessively low blood pressure
- Respiratory: Wheezing, shortness of breath, spasm of bronchial tree
- Gastrointestinal: Diarrhea, nausea, dry mouth, constipation, flatulence

ACE Inhibitors (Angiotensin Converting Enzyme)

Description

Specific competitive inhibitors of a natural hormone from the kidney named angiotensin I, a converting enzyme responsible for the conversion of angiotensin I to angiotensin II, a potent vasoconstrictor, stimulates aldosterone secretion from adrenal cortex, thereby contributing to sodium and fluid retention which leads to hypertension. This means the drugs poison the systems which make important hormones from the kidneys and the adrenals to regulate blood vessel size and blood flow to the brain. These drugs also injure other vital organs and the mineral balance in the blood and tissues.

Conventional Prescription Names

Altace, Capoten, Capozide, Lotensin, Monopril, Vasotec, Zestril, Zestoretic, Prinivil, Prinzide

Warnings

General: Massive swelling involving extremities, face, lips, mucous membranes, tongue, glottis and larynx

Blood Forming Organs: Low white blood cell count, agranulocytosis, (failure to form an essential type of white

162 blood cell in the bone marrow), anemia and thrombocytopenia (low platelets which have to do with blood clotting), can all occur. All of these conditions are severe and disabling problems with the blood cell forming organs.

Metabolic: Can cause dangerously high potassium levels, excessively low blood pressure, loss of taste and smell and kidney damage with protein loss in the urine.

Adverse Reactions
- •Cardiovascular: Cardiac arrest, strokes, fainting
- •Respiratory: Bronchospasm, inflammation of nose, shortness of breath
- •Dermatologic: Rash, pruritus (itching without a rash)
- •Gastrointestinal: Pancreatitis
- •General: Weakness, gynecomastia (enlarged male breasts)
- •Hematologic: Anemia, both aplastic and hemolytic
- •Hepatobiliary: Jaundice, hepatitis
- •Nervous/Psychiatric: Clumsiness or disuse of extremities, depression, insomnia
- •Senses: Blurred vision
- •Genitourinary: Impotence, kidney damage with loss of protein in the urine

Diuretics

Description
These drugs cause the urine to be diluted by excessive water because the kidney mechanism that reabsorbs water from the urine as it is being manufactured by the kidney is poisoned by the drug.

Conventional Prescription Names:
Aldactazide, Aldoril, Capozide, Combipres, Corzide, Diupres, Diazide, Esimil, Hydropres, Hydromox, Inderide, Lasix, Lozol, Minizide, Normozide, Serapes, Esidrix.

Warnings

Hydrochlorothiazide affects the kidney's mechanism for preventing minerals from being lost in the urine. Thiazides increase the loss of sodium and chloride by poisoning the kidney's mechanism for conserving nutrients. By the same mechanism excessive loss of potassium and magnesium may occur, and decreased tissue levels may persist even with supplementation. The risk of life-threatening arrhythmias is markedly increased by low tissue levels of potassium and magnesium. Thiazides may also cause pancreatitis, jaundice, nausea, vomiting, vertigo, dizziness, restlessness, muscle spasms, light sensitivity, and the death of tiny blood vessels with inflammation and fever.

Adverse Reactions

• Cardiovascular: Heart rhythm disturbances, fainting, excessively slow heart rate
•Respiratory: Shortness of breath, nosebleed, nasal congestion
•Gastrointestinal: Nausea, vomiting, diarrhea, loss of appetite, dry mouth, over secretion of saliva and digestive juices
•Metabolism: Weight gain, breast engorgement in men and women
•Neurologic: Parkinsonian syndrome, paradoxical anxiety, drowsiness, mental dullness
•Nervous/Psychiatric: Mental depression possibly leading to suicide
•Genitourinary: Impotence, painful urination

One of the important hazards of hypertension is an increased risk of strokes. People take medications in an effort to reduce this risk. Many are unaware that the medications above come with such serious side effects. We believe much

164 more effort should be put into finding ways to treat hypertension other than with drugs known to be hazardous to your health and life. One such piece of research was reported recently, that the risk of strokes from any cause can be reduced by eating 10 or 12 walnut halves daily or a small serving (half a cup more or less) of cooked soybeans. The essential fatty acid alpha-linolenic acid acts as an independent agent to reduce risk.[136] Popular demand could turn research into a different channel and get much more effective methods of treating hypertension.

Adrenergic Blockers, Peripheral

Description: These agents appear to work by selectively inhibiting the alpha-1 subtype of alpha adrenergic receptors, or by blockade of post-synaptic alpha-adrenoreceptors, which causes dilation of arterioles.

Conventional Prescription Names: Cardura, Dibenzyline, Esimil, Hylorel, Hytrin, Ismelin, Minipress, Minizide

Warnings: Marked hypotension in the upright position, with syncope and loss of consciousness. Dosages must be titrated very slowly and carefully.

Adverse Reactions: Postural effects, malaise/fatigue, heart rate disturbances, hypotension, edema, dizziness, somnolence, dyspnea, anxiety, insomnia.

Angiotensin II Receptor Antagonists

Description: This new agent is an angiotensin II receptor antagonist. It works as a vasodilator by blocking the vasoconstrictor effects of the vasoactive hormone, angiotensin II.

Conventional Prescription Names: Cozaar, Hyzaar (Others are in the works)

Warnings: Not to be used in pregnancy! Can cause injury or death of developing fetus!

Adverse Reactions: Muscle cramps, dizziness, insomnia, nasal congestion, angioedema, occasional elevation of liver function tests.

commentary from the authors

Both medical research and medical practice are moving targets. A major reason medical authorities and educators are so insistent upon having recent references is that research and practice change so rapidly, often abruptly. We have tried to present in this book natural, physiological methods of controlling hypertension that are, for the most part, timeless and changeless, as they are based upon human anatomy and physiology. However, we recognize that not all change is bad, and that new information is constantly being offered. The problem is to sort out that which will stand the test of time and practice. The goal is to discard that which is the latest therapeutic fad, which may prove to be not only a hindrance in the long run, but harmful.

One might get the idea from the body of information in this book that we are therapeutic nihilists. That is not the case, as we treat vigorously and carefully, although we feel we must warn the public about the hazards of indiscriminate and excessive drug use, and even the problems that may be associated with their very careful use.

In the "natural," or lifestyle-oriented method of treating hypertension that we have suggested in this book, it has been found over the past 30 years that 80-90% of hypertensives will respond favorably. The response is usually prompt, often within days or at least a few weeks. This fact has been shown in all lifestyle programs, including our own at Uchee Pines Institute, as well as those such as Wildwood, in Georgia; Poland Spring in Maine; Eden Valley in Colorado; Weimar Institute in California; the Lifestyle Center of America in Oklahoma; the Pritikin Centers, and Dean Ornish's programs based in California.

Nevertheless, around 10% remain who make a slow or incomplete response to the lifestyle methods. These may include a very few with organic causes, such as unilateral kidney arterial narrowing; various forms of serious kidney disease; adrenal gland or sympathetic nervous system tumors; and others even more unusual. But most of the incomplete responders are merely the more complex cases that still fall into the category of "essential hypertension," meaning that there is no currently recognized cause for their increased blood pressure.

What about the small number in the above group who maintain a significantly elevated blood pressure in spite of our best efforts? We would advise that the patient continue faithfully the lifestyle changes, which after all are physiological and required to maintain healthy bodies in general. They should then urgently and persistently study their lifestyles for hidden or ignored deviations from the basic health laws. Such things as overwork with insufficient rest, overeating (not much food is required to maintain ideal weight), hidden causes of stress, failure to examine labels carefully for sodium sources—all or any of these may be a culprit. Sometimes such simple measures as getting a regular full-body massage or relaxing hydrotherapy will be successful in restoring proper blood pressures.

Patients need to be aware that hypertension is a major risk factor for strokes and heart attacks, as well as congestive

167

heart failure and kidney failure. Our goal should be to pre-
serve these vital organs where possible, by controlling the
blood pressure. In the past two or three years, studies have
come out that indicate heart attack risk is definitely decreased
in those whose blood pressures are well controlled—at least
under 160-170/95-98. And studies have been available for
years showing the marked decrease in strokes for each 10
point reduction in blood pressure.

Even the newer drugs coming out currently, that are
touted as being quite safe, often have side effects that may
not be recognized before the drugs are marketed. It took almost thirty years of use to discover that the diuretics had serious drawbacks. The early total sympathetic blockers in
vogue over 30 years ago were found to cause the unacceptable side effect of fatal pulmonary fibrosis. And one has only
to recall the recent furor over the short-acting calcium-chan-
nel blockers, with the evidence of significantly increased risk
of heart attacks, to make us quite wary.

So, it would certainly behoove us to make every attempt
to control hypertension with simple, physiological methods
rather than launching out upon the largely unknown sea of
polypharmacy.

Concise Summary of Major Points of This Book To
summarize the lifestyle interventions we have suggested in
this book:

1. Reduce if overweight! Remember, although it is surely
desirable to try to attain the ideal weight, studies show that
reduction of as little as 10-15 pounds, if kept off, can be of
significant value.

2. Exercise, exercise, exercise! This need not be violent,
but should be regular, preferably daily, and out of doors. We
have a friend whose blood pressure is poorly responsive, but
will regularly drop 20-30 points systolic, and up to 10 diastolic, after a brisk jog. Another middle-aged lady keeps her
difficult-to-control blood pressure in check by the gardening

and yard work she does six days a week, and a three mile walk on the seventh day.

3. *Reduce sodium (salt) in the diet.* Use less than a gram a day until the blood pressure has been well below 140/90 for at least a week. Then one may carefully try a measured half-teaspoonful of added salt daily. If the blood pressure starts to rise again, the salt should be eliminated for a longer period, up to three months, before trying again.

4. *Eliminate visible fats from the diet.* Saturated (hard, mostly animal) fats especially must be removed. Of course, we feel that a total vegetarian diet has many benefits of its own, and this is especially true in hypertension.

5. *Avoid chilled extremities.* Chilling can raise blood pressure by reflexively narrowing arterioles.

6. *Try to avoid stress.* For the unavoidable kind, try to minimize the effects. Two of the best methods for this are exercise, which tends to reduce the effects of stress; and an abiding trust in an all-loving Creator. Some people will need to consider changing their vocations and/or environments.

7. *Develop a strong trust in God.* Make the Bible your constant companion. "Pray without ceasing" that the Holy Spirit will show to you areas of your life where there are unresolved tensions.

All of the above should be practiced by everyone who desires to control blood pressure. If they have been done faithfully, and the pressure is still elevated, then some supplements may be of value.

1. *Magnesium.* We add this mineral first, as it is a very potent relaxer of the smooth muscle lining of blood vessels, and a number of studies have shown that most people with hypertension and/or heart disease have a total body deficiency of magnesium. We find that magnesium-potassium aspartate is one of the better preparations, since potassium has additional benefits in hypertension. Try starting with two capsules three times daily, taken with meals, which enhances

absorption. An alternative is magnesium citrate, which is the best absorbed of the magnesium salts. If diarrhea occurs (unusual in the small amounts used here), reduce the dosage.

2. *Garlic.* On the whole, garlic has been somewhat disappointing, perhaps because too much has been expected of it. We like the cold-aged, deodorized product, *Kyolic.* Probably most people do not take enough. We start with two capsules of the *Superformula 102* three times a day. If response is inadequate, we either double the dose, or go to the *Kyolic Reserve,* two caps three times daily; it is roughly double the strength of the *Superformula 102.*

3. *Various herbal products.* The first one that we usually add is hawthorn berry; after that, *Coleus forskohlii* may be one of the best. There is significant foreign literature that suggests benefit in hypertension as well as asthma. Others are mistletoe (the European variety, which is not toxic in any usual dosage); dandelion leaf and root; and ginkgo biloba leaf. Literally dozens of herbal preparations have been used in hypertension; sometimes one combination will work for a specific person, and another for someone else.

4. *Flaxseed oil.* This is the highest known source of the beneficial omega-3 fatty acids. They are precursors of beneficial hormonal substances called "prostaglandins," which help to prevent smooth muscle spasm, and dilate blood vessels.

5. *L-arginine.* This free-form amino acid is the precursor of nitric acid, which has been found to be the "endothelial relaxing factor." It relaxes blood vessels markedly, but with a rather short effect. It may be tried in an amount of one gram (1000 mg) three times daily at least 1 hour before meals. The long-term effect of taking this free amino acid is not known.

We believe that careful adherence to this program will reward the person with many enhancements to his health program, including, for most, excellent control of hypertension.

170

appendix

Recommended Dietary Allowances for adults who are 23 to 50 years of age

Milligrams/day (Unless Noted)

	Men	Women
Boron	1.5-3	1.5-3
Chromium (mcg/day)	50-200	50-200
Copper	1.5-3	1.5-3
Fluoride	1.5-4	1.5-4
Iodine(mcg/day)	150	150
Iron	7-10	7-15
Magnesium	350	280
Manganese	2-5	2-5
Molybdenum(mcg/day)	75-250	75-250
Selenium (mcg/day)	70	55
Zinc	15	12

Boron

Boron has multiple functions in the human body. One well-known action of boron is in prevention and treatment of osteoporosis in women. It is used to good advantage in menopause syndromes. One of the important functions of boron is to stabilize other minerals. Copper has such a good function in making a healthy heart, and boron is essential to stabilize copper. Boron also has an important balancing relationship with magnesium. It is useful in building good muscles, keeping brain waves normal, increasing efficiency of fuel burning, and normalizing vitamin D and testosterone levels. Excellent food sources of boron include nuts, seeds, legumes, leafy vegetables, most all vegetables, apples, pears, grapes, most all fruits and their juices.

Calcium

Calcium also helps to lower blood pressure. Foods high in calcium are dry beans and peas, whole grains, greens, figs, sesame seeds and broccoli. Milk is not as good a source of calcium because of its high fat, high salt and high phosphate content, all of which the hypertensive person should avoid.

Chromium

This mineral, along with zinc and manganese, is very active in the work of the pancreas, the two latter named minerals assisting in the production of insulin, and chromium helping in the blood sugar control of the pancreas, actually getting glucose into cells. Persons who lack chromium are likely to get high blood sugar. Persons with diabetic neuropathy improve with a diet high in chromium. A high sugar content of food causes losses of chromuim in the urine.

We need at least 50 micrograms of chromium a day. Most Americans with their refined get about half that amount. Food sources include Brewers yeast, whole grain cereals and breads, herbs and legumes.

Copper

A little-studied nutrient is copper, especially considering its importance in human health. This nutrient helps prevent hardening of the arteries and heart disease. It interacts with zinc, and large doses of zinc can block absorption of copper. It is essential for the absorption and transport of iron, and anemia can result from deficiency.

A deficiency of copper can cause high blood pressure by causing a failure to release an arterial relaxing factor. Copper deficiency can also cause reduced ability of the body to dissolve microscopic clots, which could cause buildup of a clot to disastrous proportions, especially in persons with atherosclerosis or atrial fibrillation. Further, copper deficient men had lower levels of protective antioxidant enzymes, especially if the diet were high in fructose sweeteners. Good dietary sources of copper include nuts, seeds, whole wheat and all whole grains, cherries, carob beans, and all other legumes.

Iron

If the iron level is too high in the blood, the blood pressure may go up. The hemoglobin and serum iron should be maintained on the low side of normal. For women the hemoglobin level should be between 10.5-12.5, for men, between 12-14. Serum iron should ideally be kept between 20-75. If these levels are too high, it may be beneficial to donate blood regularly to the Red Cross until down to an ideal level.

Magnesium

For decades Epsom salts (magnesium sulfate) has been used as a safe and effective treatment for high blood pressure in pregnancy. It is also good for any patient with high blood pressure. Its major problem is its ability to cause loose stools if you get too much. In overdosage, the sign is that diarrhea may result. Then you must simply reduce the amount you are taking. Magnesium deficiency has been associated with a number of diseases, including high blood pressure, diabetes, heart rhythm disturbances and heart attacks.

Certain common eating habits such as drinking soft drinks, eating junk food, using excess salt and sugar also lead to magnesium loss in the urine.

Food sources of magnesium include anything with the

174 green color of chlorophyll, as it contains this mineral. That includes green leafy vegetables, cucumbers, green peas, etc. Other major food sources include whole grains, nuts, legumes, carob (a chocolate substitute), and molasses. Some fruits supply modest but significant amounts of magnesium--bananas, grapes, berries (raspberries, loganberries, blackberries, blueberries), avocado, cantaloupe and citrus. Animal products are rather poor sources of magnesium.

Myoinositol

This is a muscle sugar, closely related to glucose. It improves nerve function and is helpful in alleviating diabetic neuropathy. It is stored in the brain, heart and skeletal muscles. Good sources of myoinositol are citrus fruits, especially grapefruit; legumes, especially peanuts and dried beans; melons, especially cantaloupe; whole grains; yeast; wheat germ; blackstrap molasses; nuts.

Diabetics somehow lose large amounts of myoinositol in the urine. It promotes body production of lecithin, which is a part of nerve cells. This may account for the nerve involvement in diabetics. Coffee and its relatives--tea, colas and chocolate--deplete the body stores of myoinositol.

Potassium

Potassium acts as a major regulator of the blood pressure. Foods high in potassium are bananas, potatoes, kidney beans, peas, oranges and dried fruits. The regular eating of these foods can actually decrease blood pressure by 5-15 points.

Purines

Foods high in protein are often high in purines as well. Animal products, generally, and yeast are especially high in purines, with beans the next highest. If uric acid is high, omit all animal products, eat no more than one-half cup of beans per meal until the uric acid level falls below five on your laboratory report. Animal products and yeast can be left out of the diet entirely without causing any nutrient deficiency, except possibly vitamin B-12 in susceptible persons.

Selenium

Cancer rates are somehow related to selenium. In geographic areas where selenium blood levels are highest, cancer rates are lowest. Selenium has antioxidant and anti-inflammatory properties. It is known to stimulate the immune system. It also binds cadmium and mercury rendering them nontoxic. Yet, one can get too much selenium and develop rashes, hair loss, fatigue, dizziness, fingernail tenderness and nausea and vomiting.

A diet having abundant whole foods from plant sources should furnish plenty of selenium. The best food sources are whole grain breads and cereals, Brazil nuts, cashews, onions and many vegetables, depending on the selenium content of the soil.

Taurine

This is an amino acid-like compound which has a number of important functions in the body. It is a promoter of brain development in the unborn fetus and small child. For this use mother's milk is a good source of taurine, cow's milk a very poor source. Children whose mothers take in generous quantities of taurine in the prenatal period, and breast feed, test about five I.Q. points higher than children not having this advantage.

Taurine is useful not only in development of nerves in the young, but it has functions in regeneration of nerves as well. When nerves or brain are damaged by trauma or toxicity, it makes sense to take a diet high in taurine for its effect on regeneration of nerve tissue. Critically injured persons usually have very low blood levels of taurine while they are

176 recovering, indicating the body is using up stored taurine. Ref. *European Journal of Clinical Nutrition* 60:203-6; 1994

Another of the functions of taurine is with nerve transmission, as can be seen in its usefulness in helping to regulate heartbeat and reduce blood pressure. It functions both from its influence on nerve trunks and the tension on major muscle groups, as well as on the nerve meshworks in the walls of the arteries and arterioles where the ultimate control of blood pressure is located.

Food sources for taurine are peas, especially chick peas (garbanzos), pigeon peas and field peas; beans, notably pintos, lentils, great northern and limas; yeasts such as food or seasoning yeast and baker's yeast; and nuts and seeds, including almonds, chestnuts, cashews, pecans, walnuts, sunflower seed and sesame seed. The higher the plant food in protein, the greater the likelihood the taurine content will also be high. Carob, a healthful chocolate substitute, is high in taurine; so are whole grains. Taurine can be produced in the body from two amino acids, cysteine and methionine. Inadequate taurine causes a reduction in the flow of bile, a condition of the liver which could cause an increase in cholesterol and liver function.

Tyramine

Because of its actions to stimulate the sympathetic nervous system, the flight or fight division of the nervous system, tyramine is classed as a tension producer called a sympathomimetic amine. Other chemicals having a stronger, but similar effect are adrenalin, Neo-Synephrine, nicotine, and many drugs used in surgery to elevate the blood pressure if it should fall during a surgical procedure, such as Levophed.

Tyramine can act to raise blood pressure, promote migraine headaches, cause anxiety or sleeplessness and increase your risk of such afflictions as urinary retention, glaucoma, and muscle twitches or spasm.

Tyramine acts by releasing stored catecholamines, a form
of stress hormone. Tyramine interacts with many blood pressure medicines, notably the monoamine oxidase inhibitors
(Marplan, Niamid, Nardil, Parnate, etc.). Foods containing
large amounts of tyramine are prohibited while one is taking
those kinds of drugs.

Rich sources of tyramine in foods include hard and soft
dairy cheeses, yogurt, cottage cheese, cream cheese and buttermilk. Alcoholic drinks are also rich sources of tyramine.

178

1. Journal of the American Medical Association, 265(24): 3301, June 26, 1991
2. American Family Practitioner, June 1979, p. 177
3. Science News, 142:138, December 5, 1992
4. New England Journal of Medicine, 329:1912-1917
5. Pediatrics, 65(5):1055, May 1980
6. Patient Care, September 30, 1980, p. 33
7. Journal of the American Medical Association, 223(12):1403, March 19, 1973
8. Practical Cardiology, 9(11):118, October 1983
9. Journal of the American College of Nutrition, 12(5):595, 1993
10. Consultant, November 1993, p.36
11. Practical Cardiology, 9(11):123, October 1983
12. Modern Medicine, December 1983, p.51
13. Patient Care, September 30, 1980, p.17
14. Journal of the American Medical Association, 248:1996-2003, 1982
15. San Francisco Examiner, September 1982
16. Journal of the American Medical Association 249:2792, 1983
17. Emergency Medicine, 15(18):54, 1983
18. New England Journal of Medicine, 321:868-873, 1989
19. American Journal of Epidemiology, 136:446,

180   November 10, 1992
20. Journal of Clinical Investigation, 41(4):710, 1962
21. Journal of the American Medical Association,
    December 2, 1992, by Dr. W. Gordon Walker of
    Johns Hopkins
22. American Family Practitioner, February 1981,
    p.213
23. Archives of Internal Medicine, 152:1162-66, 1992
24. Medical World News, February 27, 1984, p.106
25. Primary Cardiology, February 1980, p.41
26. Health facts, "Hypertension Treatment: More Aggres-
    sive in the United States to no Advantage." September
    1989, p.3
27. American Journal of the Medical Sciences,
    306:345, November, 1993
28. Cell, October 2, 1992, Jean-Marc Lalouel of
    Howard Hughes Medical Institute
29. Archives of Internal Medicine, 153:290, February
    8, 1993
30. American Journal of Surgery, 165:61, January
    1993
31. Diabetologia, 35:1140, December 1992
32. Journal of Clinical Endocrinology, 37:2, August,
    1992, pp.147-55
33. The American Journal of the Medical Sciences,
    306(5):345-347, November 1993
34. Journal of the American Medical Association,
    69:104, January 6, 1993
35. American Journal of Clinical Nutrition, 38:879-
    883, 1983
36. American Journal of Hypertension, 5:585-591,
    1992, by H.G. Preuss
37. Journal of the American Medical Association,
    266:2098, November 16, 1991
38. Hypertension, 21:129-135, 1993

39. Journal of Clinical Medicine, 33:1523-9, August
     1992
40. Journal of Internal Medicine, 227:273-278, 1990,
     by K. Landin
41. Journal of Clinical Pharmacology, 32:549-535,
     1992, by J.R. Sowers
42. Journal of Clinical Investigation, 90:24-9, July 1992
43. Medical Digest, "Hiding Woes Hurts Heart," August
     15, 1992
44. Journal of Psychosomatic Research, 37(6):653-659,
     1993
45. Journal of Psychosomatic Medicine, 56:147-180,
     1994
46. Journal of Psychosomatic Research, 37(6):603-613,
     1993
47. Prodigy (R) Interactive Personal Service, August 8,
     1992
48. Dr. Jonathan Shedler, Lecture presented at the Institute
     of Advanced Psychological Studies at Adelphi Univer-
     sity in Garden City, New York; Annual Meeting of the
     American Psychological Association, August 1992
49. Biological Psychiatry 17(11):1347, 1982
50. IMAGE:Journal of Nursing Scholarship, 25:17-21,
     Spring 1993
51. British Medical Journal, 300:1368-1372; 1990
52. Medical News, Monday, February 20, 1984, p.3
53. The Physiology and Pathology of Exposure to
     Stress by Hans Selye, p.570, Montreal, Canada,
     Medical Publishers, 1950
54. Lancet, July 12, 1980, p. 60
55. Israeli Journal of Medical Science, 16(1):41-43,
     January 1980
56. The Journal of Nervous and Mental Disease,
     168(9):526-534, September 1980
57. Science News, 119:198, March 28, 1981

182

58. Lancet, November 5, 1977, p.974
59. Medical Tribune, May 23, 1979
60. Nature, January 21, 1961
61. Hydrotherapy, Gertrude Brentano Finnesty, New York, Frederick Ungar Publishing Company, p.205
62. Journal of the American Medical Association, 183(10):845
63. Ralph DeFronzo, Professor of Medicine and Chief of Diabetes at the University of Texas, Health Science Center, San Antonio; manuscript from private office
64. Angiology, 24:472-9, September 1973
65. Lancet, January 19, 1980 p.120
66. Tohoku Journal of Experimental Medicine, 72:237-242, 1960
67. Circulation, 12:963-73, December 1955
68. Heart and Lung, 9(2):306, March- April, 1980
69. British Medical Journal, October 27, 1956, p.974
70. The American Journal of Medicine, 70(6):1195, June 1981
71. Science News, 143:186, 1993
72. Postgraduate Medicine, Volume 21:67, 1957, p.67
73. Food Insight, Published by IFIC Foundation, Washington, DC, May 1994
74. Cardiovascular Reviews and Reports, Volume 3, Number 3, March 1982
75. Modern Medicine, December 1983, p.110
76. Journal of the American Medical Association, 139:685-688, March 12, 1949
77. Eat For Strength, Oil-Free Edition, Agatha M. Thrash, M.D., NewLifestyle Books, 30 Uchee Pines Road, Suite 15, Seale, AL 36875
78. The Journal of Pediatrics, 94:1012, 1979
79. Patient Care, September 30, 1980, p.33
80. Consultant, November 1993, p.36
81. Experimental Medicine in Surgery, 14(4):286-98,

1956

82. Lancet, January 8, 1983, p.8
83. British Medical Journal, September 24, 1977, p.805
84. Ibid.; (2)1541-1543, 1979
85. Proceedings of the Society for Experimental Biology in Medicine, 165:283- 290, 1980
86. Journal of the American College of Nutrition, 12(5):595, 1993
87. Postgraduate Medicine, "Magnesium Deficiency and Diabetes" 92(5):217, October 1992
88. Ibid.; 92(5):217, October 1992
89. Journal of Nutrition and Biochemistry, 1:542, October, 1990
90. Circulation, 86:1475-84, November 1992
91. Internal Medicine News, 16(20):55, October 1983
92. Ibid.; 17(3):53, February 1984
93. Science News, 142:340, November 21, 1992
94. Archives of Environmental Health, January-February, 1981, p.28-32
95. Endocrinology, 132:652, 646, February 1993
96. Journal of the American Medical Association, 237(3):262, January 17, 1977
97. Metabolism, 28(12):1234-8, December 1979
98. Archives of Internal Medicine, 143:2099-2102, 1983
99. Japanese Heart Journal, 20(5):741, September 1979
100. Biochemical Pharmacology, 27:2689-2692, 1978
101. Science News, May 1992, p.319
102. Cosmopolitan, November 1992, p.74
103. New England Journal of Medicine, 320:1037-1043, 1989
104. Consumer Reports, May 1992
105. British Medical Journal, December 15, 1979, p. 1541
106. Health and Home, 17(3):32, March 1976
107. Journal of the American Medical Association, No-

184
vember 14, 1903, p.1229

108. Klinische Wochenschriff, 3:624, April 1, 1924
109. Journal of the American Medical Association, October 6, 1978
110. New England Journal of Medicine, January 1978
111. Hypertension, 10:11231-11236, 1992
112. Internal Medicine News, 17(2):63, January 1984
113. Cardiology, 67:230, 1981
114. American Heart Journal, 106:316- 20, 1983
115. Medical Science Sports Exercise, 25:854-862, 1993
116. Proceedings of the Society for Experimental Biology in Medicine, 173:541-546, 1983
117. Lancet, 341:1248, 1249; May 15, 1993
118. Science News, 136:184-186, September 16, 1989
119. American Family Practitioner, 22(4):180, 1980
120. Ibid.; June 1979, p.177
121. Appetite, 17(2):161, 1991
122. Science News, "Delinquent Developments" May 1, 1993
123. Journal of the American Medical Association, 86(15):1159, 1925
124. Journal of Internal Medicine, 225:95-99, 1989
125. Podiatry, 54(3):103, March 1964
126. Eat For Strength, Oil-Free Edition, Agatha M. Thrash, M.D., NewLifestyle Books, 30 Uchee Pines Road, Suite 15, Seale, AL 36875
127. Journal of the American Medical Association, 86(15):1159, 1925
128. Journal of Internal Medicine, 225:95-99, 1989
129. Agricultural Research Service, USDA, Grand Forks, North Dakota
130. Science News, May 1, 1993; "Delinquent Developments"
131. Muscle and Fitness; September, 1992, page 50, by

James Roufs; also Science News 135:204, April 1, 1989

132. Hypertension, August-September, 1992; Report for American Heart Association by Doctors Declan Murphy and Judith Salerno of the National Institute on Aging

133. Science News, June 17, 1989

134. Journal of General Internal Medicine, 8:619-621, 1993

135. Preventive Medicine 24:378-388, 1995

136. Journal of American Medical Association, 273(20):1563; May 24, 1995

Index

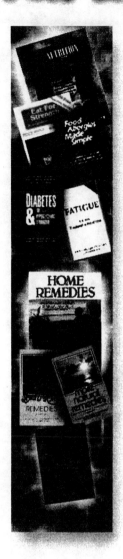